Fertility Acupuncture Handbook

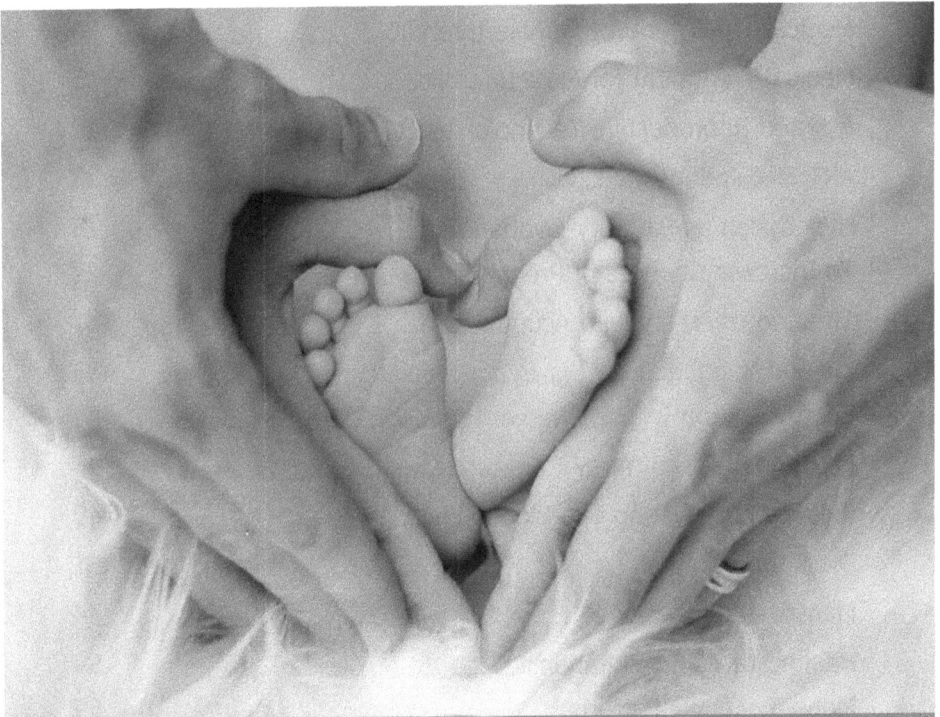

By Maurice Lavigne

Acupuncturist, Herbalist, Qi Gong Instructor & Therapist
Author of Acupuncture Diagnostic Methods &
Point Selection

TABLE OF CONTENTS

Introduction

The Fertility Acupuncture Handbook provides insight on how Traditional Chinese Medicine (TCM) teats infertility in both men and women. It details the body's energy anatomy as it relates to infertility, discusses the role of hormones in the regulation of the menstrual cycle, describes the different phases of the women's menstrual cycle, details the importance of Blood and the Heart/Uterus connection, and explores various patterns of disharmony that hinder fertility.

It offers treatment strategies to address infertility caused by a variety of conditions such as:

- Irregular Menstrual Cycle
- Blood Stasis
- Accumulation of Dampness or Cold in the Uterus
- Endometriosis
- Uterine Fibroids
- Ovarian Cysts
- Pelvic Inflammatory Disease

- Ectopic Pregnancy
- In Vitro Fertilization
- Common issues that arise in the first trimester of pregnancy
- Breached Baby
- Acupuncture Induction
- Postpartum Depression
- Low Quality Sperm

Also provided are recommendations for a healthier lifestyle, Qi Gong exercises for infertility, and diet according to the four phases of the menstrual cycle.

Fertility treatments with Traditional Chinese Medicine may:

- Improve blood flow to the reproductive organs
- Improve egg quality
- Improve ovarian function
- Stimulate ovulation
- Reduce stress levels
- Regulate the hypothalamic-pituitary-ovarian axis
- Improve hormonal production
- Normalize the menstrual cycle
- Reduce miscarriage rates
- Reduce menopause-like symptoms
  Increase rate of conception

About the Author

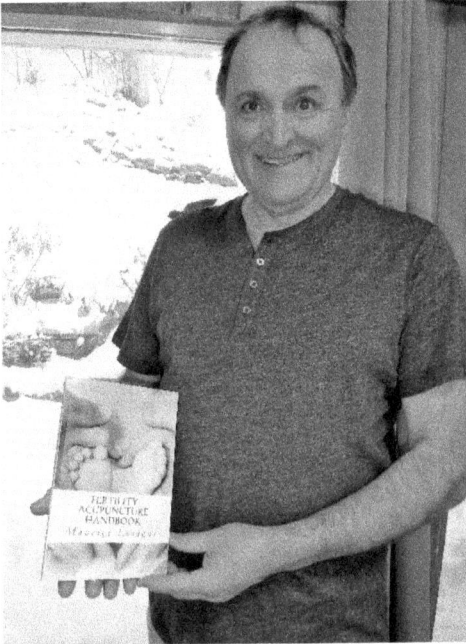

The author of this publication, Maurice Lavigne, has been offering Natural Medicine Treatments at the Fredericton Wellness Clinic located in Fredericton, New Brunswick, Canada, since 1996.

After graduating with a Bachelor of Arts Degree in Communications in 1984, he worked in Journalism, Public Relations, and Information Technology for approximately 25 years. During this time, his growing interest in Natural Medicine prompted him to explore training possibilities in complementary therapies.

Maurice obtained a Diploma in Massage Therapy in 1996, a Diploma in Acupuncture in 2009, Certification as a Qi Healer in 2008, and Certification as a Herbalist in 2013. He taught Aikido, a Japanese Martial Art, for 30 years and has been teaching Qi Gong since 1996.

In addition to this handbook on infertility, he published three books on Qi Gong, **The Power of Qi for Health and Longevity**, **Qi Gong's 5 Golden Keys,** and **Dance of the Dragon - Healing Oneself & Others,** as well as a foundational book on Acupuncture entitled **Acupuncture Diagnostic Methods and Point Selection.**

In 2015, Maurice received a plaque in recognition of his four years as President of the Maritime Association of Registered Acupuncturists (MARA). Inscribed on the Plaque**: "In Deep Appreciation of Your Talents So Generously Given."**

What is infertility?

Infertility is a condition of the reproductive system that prevents the conception of children. A diagnosis of infertility is normally given to couples who have not conceived despite regular sexual intercourse for at least one year. Infertility affects approximately 10 to 15% of couples of childbearing age.

Women are more fertile between the ages of 20 and 25. In couples younger than 30 who are generally healthy, 20% to 37% can conceive in the first 3 months. From the age of 35 there is a marked decrease in fertility.

The most significant drop in fertility is seen from the age of 38 to 39. After 39 years old, it is more difficult to conceive as there are fewer eggs, and more unnoticed miscarriages due to genetic damage.

Overall, one-third of infertility cases are caused by male reproductive issues, one-third by female reproductive issues, and one-third by both male and female reproductive issues or by unknown factors.

Essential Factors to Pregnancy

For pregnancy to occur:
- The ovaries must produce and release an egg
- The sperm must be healthy
- The couple must practice regular intercourse during fertile time
- The fallopian tubes must be free of obstruction so that the egg and sperm can meet and join.
- The Uterus must be healthy to allow for the implantation and growth of the foetus.

In healthy individuals, the process that leads to pregnancy is simple. First one of the two ovaries releases a mature egg. The egg is picked up by the fallopian tube. Sperm swim up the cervix, through the Uterus and into the fallopian tube to reach the egg for fertilization. The fertilized egg travels down the fallopian tube to the Uterus where it implants and grows. In a small percentage of couples this process does not work properly.

Causes of Infertility in Women

One of the main causes of female infertility are hormonal imbalances that lead to irregular or absent menstrual cycles, or a failure to ovulate. A woman's ovulation and menstruation are regulated by changes in certain reproductive hormones, especially estrogen.

For many women who are of reproductive age, low estrogen levels can induce missed or irregular periods, or a failure to ovulate. Hormonal imbalance can be caused by an underlying health condition, chronic stress, poor diet, too much exercise, or sudden weight gain or loss.

Irregular Menses

A normal menstrual cycle last 28 days. Abnormal cycles can be too short, too long or irregular indicating an imbalance in the reproductive system. Menstrual bleeding, which normally lasts from 3 to 5 days, is considered irregular if it occurs more frequently than every 21 days or lasts longer than 8 days.

While an irregular cycle is not always a problem, it can signal health complications and hinder efforts to conceive. In many cases, irregular menstrual cycles are related to a condition called anovulation. This means that ovulation hasn't taken place usually due to a severe hormonal imbalance.

Sometimes an irregular cycle may be due to subtler hormone imbalances. Ovulation may still occur, but the timing of the ovulation can vary greatly month to month. An irregular cycle can make it more difficult to get pregnant, especially if ovulation does not occur every month.

Ovulatory Disorders

Ovulation disorders in which ovulation fails to occur or occurs on an infrequent or irregular basis account for infertility in about 1 in 4 infertile couples.

Two hormones produced by the pituitary gland are responsible for stimulating ovulation each month – Follicle Stimulating Hormone (FSH) and Luteinizing Hormone (LH).

FSH helps control the menstrual cycle and the production of eggs by the ovaries. LH controls the length and sequence of the female menstrual cycle, including ovulation, preparation of the Uterus for implantation of a fertilized egg, and ovarian production of both estrogen and progesterone.

The production of FSH and LH can be disrupted by excess physical or emotional stress, a very high or very low body weight, or a recent substantial weight gain or loss. Irregular or absent periods are the most common signs. There are two types of ovulatory disorders: Anovulation or absence of ovulation and Oligomenorrhea or infrequent or irregular ovulation.

Anovulation is the failure of the ovary to release eggs over a period usually exceeding three months. One of the major signs of anovulation is irregular or absent menstrual periods. In anovulation, the eggs do not develop properly, or are not released from the follicles of the ovaries. Women who have this disorder may not menstruate for several months. Others may menstruate even though they are not ovulating.

Anovulation may result from hormonal imbalances, eating disorders, and other medical disorders such as Polycystic Ovarian Syndrome. Often the cause is unknown. Female athletes who exercise excessively may also stop ovulating.

Oligomenorrhea is another term for irregular but not totally absent periods, which is defined as more than 36 days between menstrual cycles or fewer than eight cycles per year.

Also called Primary Ovarian Insufficiency or Premature Ovarian Failure, this disorder is usually caused by premature loss of eggs from the ovary before age 40 possibly from chromosomal defects, an immune system response to ovarian tissue, or from toxins mainly from chemotherapy and radiation which damage genetic material in cells. If the ovaries fail, they do not produce normal amounts of estrogen or release eggs regularly. Infertility is a common result.

Follicle Stimulating Hormones (FSH) stimulate a women's ovaries to produce estrogen to begin follicular development. If the ovaries do not respond adequately, they send a message to the brain to produce more FSH. Higher levels of FSH found in the blood indicate that the ovaries may not be producing normal levels of estrogen and may be interpreted as a sign of possible ovarian failure.

The ovary no longer produces eggs, and it lowers estrogen production. Estrogen regulates the menstrual cycle. High levels of estrogen are required in the Blood for the follicles to release an egg. The low levels of estrogen trigger an increased in the production of Follicle Stimulating Hormone (FSH) which in turn increases the production of estrogen and the number of follicles.

Ovarian reserve refers to the reproductive potential available within a woman's ovaries based on the number and quality of her eggs. High levels of FSH can be an indication that the body is trying to increase a low egg supply, improve poor egg quality or counter premature menopause.

Premature Ovarian Failure is sometimes referred to as premature menopause, but the two conditions aren't the same. Women with premature ovarian failure can have irregular or occasional periods for years and might even become pregnant. Women with premature menopause stop having periods and can't become pregnant.

FSH levels can be lowered by taking synthetic estrogen and birth control pills. Lowering FSH levels does not necessarily correlate with an improvement of ovarian reserves.

Hormonal imbalances represent 40% of documented cases of infertility. Traditional Chinese Medicine is very effective in correcting hormonal imbalance. It has a long history of helping women with elevated FSH to conceive.

Through the use of acupuncture and herbs TCM improves blood flow into the reproductive organs and restores hormonal balance, often reducing FSH levels. Dietary changes and stress reduction techniques are often a critical component of the overall protocol for women with elevated FSH.

Other Hormonal Imbalances

Polycystic Ovary Syndrome (PCOS)
Polycystic Ovary Syndrome (PCOS) is a hormonal disorder common among women of reproductive age. It is associated with insulin resistance and obesity, abnormal hair growth on the face or body, and acne. It's one of the most common causes of female infertility.

Women with PCOS display higher-than-normal levels of male hormones such as testosterone. They may have difficulties getting pregnant because of irregular ovulation or failure to ovulate as the ovaries develop many fluid follicles that fail to release eggs regularly.

Luteal Phase Defect
A Luteal Phase Defect occurs after ovulation and before menses. When a suspected Luteal Phase Defect occurs, the secretion of progesterone by the ovary is below normal or the endometrium does not respond to the normal stimulation of progesterone.

During this phase of the menstrual cycle the lining of the uterus normally gets thicker to prepare for a possible pregnancy. With a Luteal Phase Defect, that lining doesn't grow properly each month. A Luteal Phase Defect is associated with both infertility and early miscarriage.

Too Much Prolactin
When the pituitary gland produces too much prolactin, it reduces estrogen production which may lead to infertility. Eggs won't mature adequately if estrogen is deficient early in the cycle. Usually this condition is related to a pituitary gland problem but can also be caused by medications being administered for another disease.

Stress
Stress leads to the release of hormones that negatively affect the menstrual cycle. Stress overstimulates the sympathetic nervous system diverting the Blood flow from the ovaries and Uterus to the adrenals which may cause irregular cycles, lack of ovulation, and infertility.

Excess Mucus
Appropriate levels of estrogen are required to thin the cervical mucus allowing the sperm to enter the uterus. Excess mucus stops the sperm from travelling through the cervix into the Uterus.

Other Causes of Infertility

Fibroids or Polyps
Common in the Uterus, fibroids or polyps can block fallopian tubes or interfere with implantation, affecting fertility. However, many women who have fibroids or polyps do become pregnant.

Endometriosis
Endometriosis occurs when tissue that normally grows in the Uterus implants and grows in other locations. This extra tissue growth, and the surgical removal of it, can cause scarring, which may block fallopian tubes and inhibit the joining of the egg and sperm.

Endometriosis can also affect the lining of the Uterus, disrupting implantation of the fertilized egg. The condition also seems to affect fertility in less-direct ways, such as damage to the sperm or egg.

Age (Decline starts at age 39)
More women are choosing to delay starting a family until later in life when their reproductive health is diminished. The quality and quantity of a woman's eggs begin to decline with age. In the mid-30s, the rate of follicle loss speeds, resulting in fewer and poorer quality eggs, making conception more difficult, and increasing the risk of miscarriage.

Sexual History
Sexually transmitted infections such as chlamydia and gonorrhea can damage the fallopian tubes. Therefore, having unprotected intercourse with multiple partners increases the risk of a sexually transmitted infection that may cause fertility problems later. In addition, antibodies used to combat cervical or vaginal infections may kill or inhibit the sperm.

Sexual Activity

Sexual activity before and during puberty is an increasingly frequent cause of infertility as it weakens the Kidneys and damages the Ren and Chong vessels which may lead to infertility later in life. In addition, sex during the period may lead to Blood Stasis, an important cause of infertility in women.

Physical Obstructions

Physical obstructions can occur in the ovaries, fallopian tubes or uterus. They can be caused by uterine abnormalities from birth, such as an abnormally shaped Uterus, Cervical Stenosis which is a narrowing of the cervix caused by an inherited malformation or damage to the cervix or scarring from surgical intervention.

Damage to the Fallopian Tubes

Damaged or blocked fallopian tubes keep the sperm from getting to the egg or block the passage of the fertilized egg to the Uterus caused by:
- Pelvic Inflammatory Disease, an infection of the Uterus and fallopian tubes due to chlamydia, gonorrhea or other sexually transmitted infections
- Previous surgery in the abdomen or pelvis, including surgery for ectopic pregnancy, in which a fertilized egg implants and develops in a fallopian tube instead of the Uterus
- Pelvic tuberculosis, a major cause of tubal infertility worldwide, although uncommon in North America.

Constitutional Deficiency

Constitutional deficiency from a premature birth, unhealthy mother, older parents, weak constitution of parents, or conception or birth complications. In Traditional Chinese Medicine, constitutional weakness is an indication of a Deficiency of Kidney Jing. As Kidney Jing forms the foundation for Tian Gui or Menstrual Blood, women suffering from Deficiency of Jing may not be able to conceive.

Weight Gain or Loss

Being overweight or significantly underweight may affect normal ovulation. Women who are overweight often suffer from Dampness and Stagnation of Qi and Blood. Extra body fat may also raise the levels of estrogen and other hormones increasing the risk of breast cancer.

Smoking
Besides damaging the cervix and fallopian tubes, smoking increases the risk of miscarriage and ectopic pregnancy. It's also thought to age the ovaries and deplete the eggs prematurely.

Alcohol
Drink no more than one alcoholic drink per day as both men and women who consume more than five alcoholic beverages a week experience lowered fertility. Alcoholic beverages contain a lot of sugar. Excessive sugar consumption decreases fertility by contributing to hormonal imbalance, insulin resistance, yeast infections, vitamin and mineral deficiency, and lowered immunity.

Overwork & Strenuous Physical Activity
Doing too much work, without taking time to recharge, along with an irregular diet is a common cause of Kidney Yin Deficiency. Kidney Yin is important in the formation of menstrual Blood, and the health of the Uterus. Strenuous sport or physical activity over a prolonged period can weaken the Spleen and Kidney Yang. This is especially critical at puberty, when the girl's Uterus is developing.

Diet
Excessive consumption of cold foods such as iced foods and drinks can lead to an invasion of pathogenic Cold with Cold obstructing the Uterus. Greasy foods and dairy products can lead to Dampness in the lower abdomen which can cause blocked fallopian tubes.

Invasion of Cold
Invasion of Cold is a common cause of infertility in young women. This condition may develop during puberty when young girls are exposed to Cold and Damp environments when exercising or playing outdoor sports especially during their period. As Cold invades the Uterus, it turns over time into internal Cold, obstructing the Uterus, and Ren and Chong Vessels preventing fertilisation.

Unexplained infertility
A combination of several minor factors in both partners could cause unexplained fertility problems. Illnesses, injuries, environmental toxins, chronic health problems, and lifestyle choices can also play a role in infertility.

Consulting a Doctor

The American Society for Reproductive Medicine recommends that a woman who is trying to conceive consult her medical doctor if she is:
1) Under 35 years old and has been trying to conceive for more than 12 months
2) Over 35 years old and has been trying to conceive for over 6 months
3) Over 40 years old

The doctor will conduct a thorough physical exam of both partners to determine their general state of health and to identify any physical disorders that may be contributing to infertility. After the first appointment, the physician may proceed with some initial testing to evaluate:
- If ovulation is occurring
- When it is occurring
- Ovarian function
- Uterine function during the ovulation process
- Quality of the sperm

A urine or Blood test may be ordered to check for infections or a hormone problem. An analysis of body temperature and cervical mucus and tissue will help determine if ovulation is occurring.

A cervical mucus test performed several hours after intercourse will help determine if the sperm is able to penetrate and survive in the cervical mucus. A tiny telescope with a fiber light may be used to look for uterine abnormalities. A laparoscope inserted into the abdomen will provide a view of the condition of the organs and help identify any blockages, adhesions or scar tissue.

An ultrasound done vaginally or abdominally will assess the thickness of the lining of the Uterus (endometrium) and monitor follicle development. Conducted two to three days after ovulation, an ultrasound will confirm whether an egg has been released. A sonohystogram combines an ultrasound with saline injected into the Uterus to look for abnormalities or other problems.

Ideally, the female patient will have already begun tracking ovulation through fertility awareness or a fertility monitor.

Medical Treatment for Female Infertility

Medical treatment for infertility in women may involve:

- Taking fertility medications or hormones to address a hormone imbalance, endometriosis, or a short menstrual cycle
- Taking fertility medications to stimulate ovulation
- Taking fertility medications to stimulate the release of the eggs
- Using supplements to enhance fertility
- Taking antibiotics to remove an infection
- Undergoing surgery to treat fallopian tube problems and endometriosis or to help remove a blockage or scar tissues from the Uterus or pelvic area.
- Surgery to retrieve eggs or sperm to be used in fertility treatments
- Reverse sterilization surgery like a vasectomy or tubal ligation

Can female infertility be prevented?

Twenty-five (25%) of infertile couples have more than one cause of infertility. Some causes of female infertility cannot be changed, such as age, family history, illness, or history of miscarriage. However, there are several things that women can do to increase fertility:

- Take steps to prevent sexually transmitted diseases
- Avoid illicit drugs and tobacco
- Avoid heavy or frequent alcohol use
- Adopt good personal hygiene, healthy diet, and a healthy lifestyle

Traditional Chinese Medicine has identified many conditions that can lead to female infertility which affect both the hormonal and menstrual cycles such as accumulation of Dampness and Phlegm, Cold in the Uterus and Kidney insufficiency.

Treatment with acupuncture and Chinese herbs focuses on strengthening the Kidney Qi and harmonizing the hormonal and menstrual cycles. This brings more Qi and Blood to the reproductive organs supporting the body's natural ability to conceive.

Medical Treatment for Male Infertility

Modern medicine offers many treatments to help address male infertility such as:
- Taking medications to help increase sperm production
- Taking antibiotics to heal an infection
- Taking hormones to improve hormone imbalance
- Taking supplements

Male infertility usually occurs because of:

1. Abnormal sperm function
- Number of sperm
- Sperm motility (Movement)
- Sperm morphology (Shape)
- Sperm liquefaction (Frees the sperm from its protective gel so transportation may occur)
- Sperm life span

2. Problems with the delivery of the sperm
- Blockage of ejaculatory ducts
- Problems with ejaculation
- A genetic disease

In about 50% of cases, the cause of male infertility cannot be determined.

Causes of Sperm Abnormality

Varicocele or a mass of varicose veins in the spermatic cord draining the testicles affects about 40% of men with infertility problems. It is the most common case of men producing less sperm than normal.

Other causes:
- Swollen veins in the scrotum
- Inflammation of the testicles
- Abnormally developed testicles
- Hernia repairs
- Hormonal disorder
- A pre-existing genetic condition

- Use of alcohol, tobacco or other drugs
- Severe mumps infection after puberty
- Complications from radiation therapy or surgery
- Exposure to poisonous chemicals or radiation
- Blockage caused from a previous infection
- Wearing restrictive or tight underwear
- Injury to the groin area
- History of Sexually Transmitted Diseases (STDs)
- Urinary tract infections
- Use of certain types of medications
- Immune responses of the body against the sperm

Ejaculation Problems May Include
- Premature ejaculation
- Retrograde ejaculation, which occurs when the semen is forced back into the bladder
- Erection dysfunctions

Tests to Assess Male Fertility

The medical doctor may proceed with the following tests to determine the origin of male infertility.

- Physical examination of the penis, scrotum and prostate
- Blood test to check for infections or hormone problems. Hormone levels are as important in male fertility as they are in female fertility.
- Taking a culture of fluid from the penis to check for infections
- Semen analysis to determine the number and quality of sperm

A semen analysis it one of the first tests done to help find out if a man has a problem fathering a child. A semen analysis measures how much semen a man produces, as well as the number and quality of sperm in the semen sample. Tests that may be done during a semen analysis include:

Volume - This is a measure of how much semen is present in one ejaculation.

Liquefaction Time - Semen is a thick gel at the time of ejaculation. It normally becomes liquid within 20 minutes after ejaculation facilitating the movement of the sperm in its search for the egg. Liquefaction time is the time it takes for the semen to turn to liquid.

Sperm Count - This counts the number of sperm present per milliliter (mL) of semen in one ejaculation.

Sperm Morphology - This is a measure of the percentage of sperm that have a normal shape.

Sperm Motility - This is a measure of the percentage of sperm that can move forward normally.

pH - This is a measure of the acidity (low pH) or alkalinity (high pH) of the semen.

White Blood Cell Count - White Blood cells are not normally present in semen.

Fructose Level - This is a measure of the amount of fructose in the semen. The fructose provides energy for the sperm.

Supporting Sperm Health

Sperm are quite sensitive and responsive to their environment. To support sperm health the male partner should:

- Follow a healthy diet
- Maintain cool scrotal temperatures. Avoid hot tubs or saunas, tight underwear, laptops on lap, taking long hot showers.
- Check for current or history of infections
- Remember that many prescription and recreational drugs can have side effects such as decreased sperm count and motility
- In men with poor quality sperm, excessive alcohol consumption is associated with a further decrease in the number of normal sperm.
- Avoid exposure to environmental contaminants and chemicals that play a significant role in decreased semen quality.

Acupuncture and herbal medicine may help some men overcome infertility problems by improving the quality of the sperm. Research has found that five weeks of acupuncture treatment reduces the number of structural abnormalities in sperm and increases the overall number of normal sperm.

According to TCM, the father gives of his essence through the sperm, temporarily losing his essence through organism and ejaculation. This can lead to a weakening of the Kidneys. Therefore, in TCM the focus on men's health is strengthening the Kidney Qi and Essence.

One-third of infertility problems are related to men. One-third involves both partners. Therefore, sperm testing is recommended for all male partners in couples seeking fertility support. At-home semen analysis kits are available to help encourage male fertility testing.

Assisted Reproductive Technologies

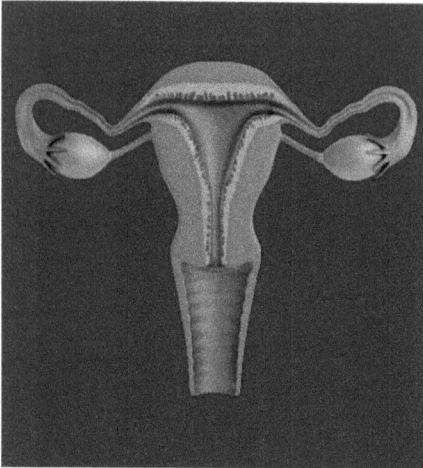

In the 1970s, British doctors began removing eggs from women who had trouble conceiving and fertilized the eggs in a laboratory. Researchers called this experimental procedure In Vitro Fertilization (IVF), and after many attempts the first test-tube baby was born in 1978.

Today, Assisted Reproductive Technology (ART) refers to all treatments that involve handling eggs or embryos outside the body. This includes IVF as well as a few of its variations. These procedures are usually paired with fertility drugs to increase success rates. About 22 percent of ART procedures result in the birth of a baby.

No long-term health effects have been linked to children born using ART procedures, but ART can be invasive and expensive. Despite the possibility of a multiple pregnancy, for many people with fertility problems ART is considered as the best chance of having a biological child.

Intrauterine Insemination (IUI)

Intrauterine Insemination is not considered an Assisted Reproductive Technology as it does not treat eggs or the embryo outside of the Uterus. Where appropriate, it is one of the fist procedures used to help with infertility as it is less invasive and less expensive than In Vitro Fertilization.

The goal of IUI is to increase the number of sperm that reach the fallopian tubes thus increasing the chance of fertilization. The most common reasons for proceeding with IUI are a low sperm count or decreased sperm mobility plus:

- Hostile cervical condition, including cervical mucus problems
- Cervical scar tissue from past procedures which may hinder the sperms' ability to enter the Uterus
- Ejaculation dysfunction
- Unexplained infertility

In preparing for IUI a nasal spray that decreases the levels of estrogen in the blood, or hormonal contraceptives such as the birth control pill may be used to prevent ovulation from naturally occurring. Fertility medications are then used to stimulate the ovaries to produce more eggs.

An ultrasound indicates if there are sufficient eggs to proceed with insemination. Fertility medications are then used to time the release of the eggs with the introduction of the sperm. A thin tube carries washed sperm directly into a woman's Uterus through the vagina.

IUI provides the sperm with a head start, but still requires it to reach and fertilize the egg on its own. Sperm is from a partner or donor when the male is infertile or when the female is single or has a same sex partner.

IUI has a 20% success rate depending mainly on the age of the female. Normally the procedure will be offered only three to six times in two-month intervals as there are diminishing returns after each failed procedure. If IUI fails, the Doctor may recommend IVF.

In Vitro Fertilization (IVF)

About 99% of ART procedures done in the United States are IVF treatments. As the name implies, IVF combines the female's eggs with the partner's sperm in a glass jar in a laboratory. After fertilization, the resulting embryos develop for three to five days before being transferred to the Uterus.

IVF is used to treat infertility in patients with ovulation disorders such as premature ovarian failure, blocked, damaged or missing fallopian tubes, uterine fibroids, male factor infertility including decreased sperm count or sperm motility issues, a genetic disorder or unexplained infertility.

In Vitro Fertilization involves many steps that allows fertilization to happen outside a woman's body.

- Suppression of the endocrine system with a drug that simulates menopause
- Fertility drugs help the woman's ovaries produce one or more eggs
- The eggs are retrieved through the vagina via needle aspiration
- A sample of sperm is provided
- Inside a lab, the eggs are fertilized in a dish with the washed sperm to produce one or more embryos.
- If successful, an embryo is transferred to the woman's Uterus through a thin tube to achieve pregnancy
- Daily progesterone injections may be provided to improve the chances of the embryos implanting successfully.

The number of embryos transferred typically depends on the number of eggs collected and maternal age of the female. The rate of implantation decreases as women age. Therefore, more eggs may be implanted in older women. The greater number of eggs transferred, the increased chances of having multiple pregnancies.

IVF is never the first step in the treatment of infertility. Instead, it's reserved for cases in which other methods such as fertility drugs, surgery, and artificial insemination haven't worked.

Possible side effects after IVF may include passing a small amount of fluid after the procedure, mild cramping or bloating, constipation and breast tenderness.

Egg retrieval carries risks of bleeding, infection, and damage to the bowel or bladder. There is also a risk of multiple pregnancies which can lead to premature delivery and low birth weight. Most women can resume normal activities the day following the procedure.

The rates of miscarriage are similar to unassisted conception, but the risk does increase with maternal age. Normally an ectopic pregnancy happens in 2% of natural pregnancies. The risk of ectopic pregnancy with IVF is 2 to 5%.

Almost all ectopic pregnancies occur in the fallopian tube and are thus sometimes called tubal pregnancies. They are often the result of an infection or inflammation of the fallopian tube, scar tissue from a previous infection or surgical procedure, and abnormal growths or birth defects.

IVF may lead to more severe symptoms in cases of OHSS (Ovarian Hyperstimulation Syndrome) which presents as swollen and painful ovaries often caused by the injection of too much hormone medication.

Other symptoms may include rapid weight gain, abdominal pain, blood clots in the legs, vomiting and shortness of breath may ensue. Women with this condition should contact their doctor right away especially if they develop breathing problems or leg pain.

The success of IVF depends on many factors including reproductive history, maternal age, the cause of infertility, and lifestyle factors. For example, women with mechanical fertility issues like fallopian tube obstruction are more likely to give birth than those with unexplained infertility or ovulatory issues.

In the United States, the live birth rate for each IVF cycle is approximately:

41-43% for women under age 35
33-36% for women ages 35 to 37
23-27% for women ages 38 to 40
13-18% for women ages over 40

In 2010, 11,806 IVF treatments were performed at Canada's 28 IVF centers which resulted in 3,188 live births, a success rate of 27%. (Source: Canadian Assisted Reproductive Technologies Registry - CARTR)

Please note that live birth rates are not the same as pregnancy rates.

IVF is expensive, and many insurance plans do not provide coverage for fertility treatment. The cost for a single IVF cycle can range from $12,000 to $17,000.

ART Medications

Medications are a regular and normal part of infertility treatments and In Vitro Fertilization (IVF) to prepare the body for treatment and increase the probability that more healthy eggs are released from the ovaries. Most hormonal medications prescribed during ART are designed to increase production of eggs but do not improve the quality of the eggs.

Some of the fertility medications used are:

Follicle Stimulating Hormone (FSH) to directly stimulate growth of the follicles.

Human Menopausal Gonadotropins (hMG) to stimulate the ovaries to produce multiple eggs during one cycle.

Synthetic Human Chorionic Gonadotropin (hCG) to trigger ovulation.

Clomiphene Citrate (CC) to stimulate ovulation in women who have absent periods, infrequent periods or long cycles.

Gonadotropin-Releasing Hormone (GnRH) to stimulate the pituitary gland to secrete LH and FSH. (Luteinizing Hormones trigger ovulation and the development of the corpus luteum.)

Progesterone to thicken the uterine lining and prepare the body to support the embryo, so the embryo will successfully implant and grow. Progesterone supplements are provided until the placenta can generate sufficient amounts.

According to some practitioners, progesterone therapy after ovulation is the only good Western therapy to help implant the egg. In TCM the strategy is to regulate the period first then promote progesterone by boosting Jing and Blood.

Fertility Supplements: Many couples opt for natural, non-prescription fertility supplements containing vitamins, minerals, antioxidants and herbs to help improve their reproductive health.

Possible Side Effects

Some medications have no known side effects. Other may present some of the following:
- Hot flashes
- Headaches
- Blurred vision
- Nausea
- Dizziness
- Nasal congestion
- Mood swings and depression
- Insomnia
- Vaginal dryness
- Decreased breast size
- Painful intercourse
- Bone density loss
- Mild hyperstimulation which includes enlarged ovaries, abdominal pain, and bloating
- Decreased Blood pressure
- Increased incidence of miscarriage, multiple births, and premature delivery
- Breast tenderness, swelling, or rash at injection site
- Ovarian cysts and pelvic discomfort from over stimulation of the ovaries

Hypothalamic, Pituitary, Ovarian Axis

The Hypothalamic–Pituitary–Ovarian Axis refers to the Hypothalamus, Pituitary Gland, and Ovaries as if they were a single system. HPO plays a critical part in the development and regulation of the reproductive and immune systems. Fluctuations in this axis cause changes in the hormones produced by each gland which may have various local and systemic effects on the body.

The hypothalamus is the regulatory control center for all hormonal activity. It secrets Gonadotropin-Releasing Hormone (GnRH) which governs ovulation, menstruation, pregnancy and sperm production. The GnRH stimulates the anterior lobe of the pituitary gland to secrete:

- Follicle-Stimulating Hormone (FSH) which stimulates the growth and maturation of eggs in the ovary.

- Luteinizing Hormone (LH) which stimulates ovulation and the development of the corpus luteum in the female and the production of testosterone by the interstitial cells of the testis in the male.

The corpus luteum secrets progesterone, a female sex hormone which prepares the endometrium for implantation. Progesterone is later produced by the placenta during pregnancy to prevent rejection of the developing embryo or fetus. Declining progesterone and estrogen levels cause thinning of the endometrium affecting embryo implantation. Boosting Blood and Qi with acupuncture and herbal medicine will boost progesterone levels.

Progesterone heats up the Uterus and allows for ovulation. This is a natural heating up of the Uterus but it may worsen a women's condition in the presence of pre-existing Liver Qi and Blood Stagnation, which by their very nature generate Heat.

The gonads (testis or ovary) produce estrogen, the primary female sex hormone produced by the ovaries and, in lesser amounts, by the adrenal cortex, placenta, and male testes.

The gonads also produce testosterone, the primary male sex hormone also produced by the adrenal cortex in both males and females.

Testosterone stimulates the development of the male reproductive organs.

By reducing stress acupuncture stimulates the release of beta-endorphins that influence the Hypothalamic-Pituitary-Ovarian Axis improving ovarian function, thus creating more follicles and better egg production.

High levels of prolactin, the hormone that stimulates the production of breast milk, may prevent ovulation and thus pregnancy but not in all cases.

Hormone Regulation: East VS West

Fertility drugs for women can produce a 20 to 60 percent pregnancy rate. They also commonly include side effects such as abdominal tenderness, bloating, fluid retention, weight gain, and nausea. Some studies show that they may also cause breast cancer.

Acupuncture infertility treatment, by contrast, produces few or no side effects while performing the same function as the drugs stimulating the hypothalamus to effectively balance the endocrine system and its hormones.

An imbalance in reproductive hormones can also negatively affect male reproductive function, such as sperm motility and production. Fertility drugs that stimulate ovulation in women by regulating the hypothalamus and pituitary glands don't perform nearly as well for men. Success rates are about a third of those for women.

The effectiveness of male infertility treatments can be greatly enhanced with herbal medicine which normally causes no side effects.

To Increase Chances of Pregnancy

Make Sure the Body is Receptive to Pregnancy

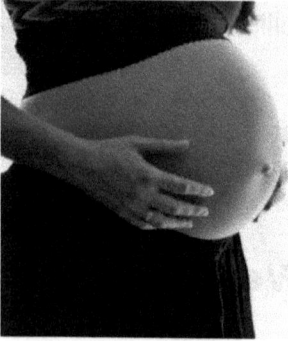

A receptive body is warm, enveloping, holding, and supportive. Spending time with pregnant women and babies helps increase receptivity to pregnancy.

Patients must not constantly expend all their energy working out or following the latest fad diet as there may not be enough energy left to support new life. Do everything in moderation.

Don't Obsess

The more emphasis put on the failure to conceive, the more stress and frustration. This in turn, may lead to more fertility hurdles. Develop a neutral attitude toward the outcome of efforts to get pregnant. Being more conscious of the process helps maintain balance and, ultimately, gives better results.

Chart the Menstrual Cycle

It is important to chart the menstrual cycle to identify any issues with ovulation, to track changes that occur because of acupuncture or herbal treatments, and to increase the chances of getting pregnant by timing sexual intercourse with the release of the egg allowing the sperm and egg to meet in the fallopian tubes.

Different Methods to Chart the Cycle

Cervical secretion is a manifestation of Kidney Jing. It occurs before ovulation at the end of the follicular phase under the influence of estrogen. It is highly predictive of ovulation and announces the beginning of the ovulation phase.

Women wishing to get pregnant should note the presence or absence of cervical secretions, checking both at midday and early evening when they are less likely to have sex. Fertile cervical secretions are clear, wet, slippery, stretching and changing in quality. They are often compared to egg whites. Infertile secretions are unchanging and generally dry, sticky, cloudy, and do not stretch.

The day of ovulation is usually the day when cervical mucus is most wet and slippery. In the days that follow that peak, especially when the cervix is dry again, fertility is at its lowest.

Charting Basal Body Temperature (BBT) identifies fertile times and confirms if, when and how smoothly ovulation is occurring. It helps determine the body's overall reproductive health by tracking ovulation, and the length and stability of the different phases of the menstrual cycle.

The average body temperature is 98.6°F (37°C). Some studies have shown that the body temperature can range from 97 to 99°F (36.1 to 37.2°C).

The BBT is taken while in bed in the morning before getting up after a minimum of four hours of relatively uninterrupted sleep. Before ovulation the optimal temperature ranges from 97.2 to 97.8°F (36.2 to 36.6°C). After ovulation the temperature ranges from 97.8 to 98.6°F (36.6 to 37°C). A typical graph will show a slight drop in temperature just prior to ovulation of about 0.3°F followed by a rise of about 0.5°F or higher reflecting the rise in progesterone levels following ovulation.

After ovulation, the temperature should remain elevated for 12 to 14 days and then drop indicating the onset of menses. With conception the temperature remains elevated and may even rise.

If the basal body temperature does not go down in the menstrual phase, it is a sign of Blood Stasis. A basal body temperature that remains flat in the Follicular Phase of the menstrual cycle is a sign of Kidney Yang Deficiency. If the basal body temperature goes up and down, it is a sign of Heart and Liver Fire.

The BBT graph can also reveal a disharmony of the Luteal Phase when, after ovulation, the temperature does not rise as dramatically as it should. The BBT rises, lowers and rises again pointing to problems with the corpus luteum often indicating Kidney Yang or Spleen Qi Deficiency. This pattern can also indicate obstruction from the presence of Blood Stasis or Damp Heat especially with endometriosis.

Day of Cycle	1	2	3	4	5	6	7	8	9	10	11	12	13	14	15	16	17	18	19	20	21	22	23	24	25	26	27	28	29	30	31	32	33	34
Day of Month	15	16	17	18	19	20	21	22	23	24	25	26	27	28	29	30	31	1	2	3	4	5	6	7	8	9	10	11						
Date																																		
Time																																		

most fertile days

3 days of elevated temperature means that ovulation has occurred

Temperature scale (°F): 99.1, 99.0, 98.9, 98.8, 98.7, 98.6, 98.5, 98.4, 98.3, 98.2, 98.1, 98.0, 97.9, 97.8, 97.7, 97.6, 97.5, 97.4, 97.3, 97.2, 97.1, 97.0, 96.9

| Intercourse | | | | | | | | X | X | | X | X | X | | X | | | X | | | | | | | | | | | | | | | | |
| Cervical Mucus Textures | P | P | P | P | D | D | D | S | S | S | E | E | E | E | E | S | S | S | S | S | D | D | D | D | D | D | | | | | | | | |

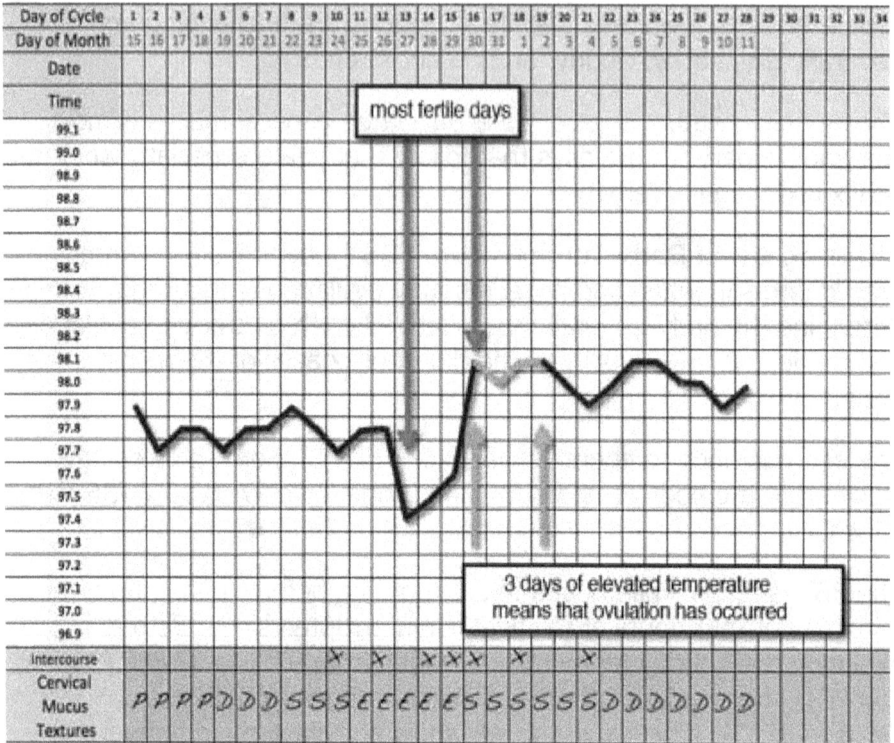

Source: zoombaby.co.uk

Ovulation Predictor Kits (OPKs)

Ovulation Predictor Kits (OPKs) provide additional confirmation on the window of fertility and can be useful for women who have just started to chart their cycle and are in the process of learning how to interpret their fertility signs. OPKs are useful for detecting impending ovulation but they can sometimes be misleading and shouldn't be relied upon alone as a means of determining fertile days. OPKs can tell you when you may be approaching ovulation, but they don't tell you if you have ovulated.

A positive ovulation test result doesn't necessarily mean it's the best time to try to conceive because without the presence of fertile cervical fluid in the vagina, the sperm is going nowhere. Bottom line, when trying to get pregnant, it is important to track cervical fluid to know when you are fertile and basal body temperature to confirm that ovulation has occurred.

The best time to try to conceive is just before ovulation. The presence of egg white or watery cervical fluid tells you it is time to have sex. The basal body temperature tells you whether ovulation has occurred.

Certain drugs can throw off the validity of OPKs. These include most fertility drugs especially those that contain Luteinizing Hormone (LH), Follicle-Stimulating Hormone (FSH), or Human Chorionic Gonadotropin (HCG), certain antibiotics, and hormone replacement therapy (HRT).

Daily Journal

In addition to tracking ovulation via BBT or OPKs, it is useful to keep a daily journal of symptoms that occur at various phases throughout the cycle. This information helps establish a more targeted treatment plan and helps track positive changes in the women's reproductive system.

Avoid dampness

Dampness accumulates in our bodies and causes blockages in the form of cysts and fibroids that can make getting pregnant difficult. When trying to become pregnant, patients must eliminate damp foods like milk, cheese, yogurt, butter, ice cream, greasy foods, and alcohol. Avoid wet clothing, humid environments, and moist basements.

Diet

Eat a healthy diet being careful to reduce intake of fatty foods, sugar, dairy products and refined foods. Focus on dark leafy green vegetables, fruits, legumes, nuts, seeds and seaweed. Organic produce is the preferred choice where possible to avoid consumption of hormones and other chemicals found in non-organic foods. Additional information on diet is provided later in this manual.

Additional Recommendations

- Avoid contact with environmental toxins
- Enjoy regular exercise
- Reduce alcoholic intake and if you smoke, quit!
- Reduce stress by practicing meditation and being physically active
- Take time away from daily activities to rest
- Practice intercourse around the ovulation cycle

Treating Infertility with Acupuncture

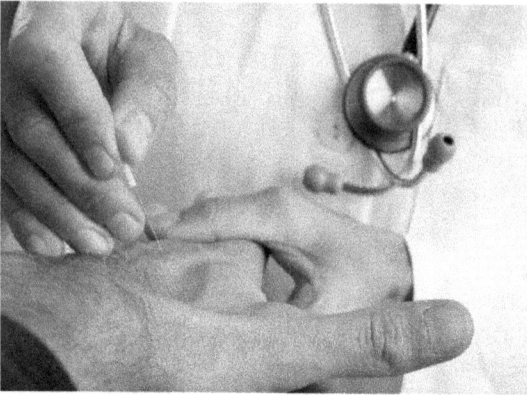

Over the past few decades, fertility rates have dropped in the Western world. To remedy the problem Western Medicine advocates the use of Intrauterine Insemination (IUI), In Vitro Fertilization (IVF) and Hormonal Therapy among other methods. Success rates with Western Medicine are not always optimal and the treatments can be invasive.

A growing number of doctors support the use of Traditional Chinese Medicine (TCM), specifically Acupuncture and Herbal Medicine, for treating infertility, as a stand-alone treatment or as a support to ART. Of all the alternative health systems, TCM appears to have the highest rate of success. With TCM the treatment must always fit the pattern and not the disease.

For centuries, TCM practitioners have helped families to conceive. Once the foundation of the body is healthy and Qi or life energy flows freely, the body is normally able to conceive. Having a baby is a priority in the Chinese culture and the TCM system for treating infertility is based on many years of accumulated experience of both patient and doctor.

For a woman to become pregnant she must produce healthy eggs and the man must produce healthy sperm. The fallopian tubes must be open to allow the sperm to reach the egg. The fertilized egg or embryo must then be able to implant successfully in the woman's Uterus. A healthy embryo and hormonal environment are required for the pregnancy to develop properly.

According to Traditional Chinese Medicine, causes of infertility begin in the Uterus. The female reproductive system in TCM consists of the Uterus, which includes the fallopian tubes and the ovaries, the cervix, birth canal, vaginal orifice and the surrounding meridians or energy pathways.

The Uterus, also called the "Child's Palace", lies in the Lower Abdomen, in the center of pelvic cavity, behind the Urinary Bladder and in front of the rectum. Its lower opening connects with the birth canal.

The Uterus is one of the six Extraordinary Yang Organs with the Marrow, Brain, Bone, Vessels and Gallbladder. Its primary function is to produce menses and cultivate the fetus. To function properly, it needs a rich supply of Qi, Blood, and Essence.

Its Yang aspect is reflected in the fact that it is hollow and stores Blood. Its role is to fill and discharge. It discharges Blood from the Uterus, ova from the ovaries, and the mature fetus from the Uterus at the end of pregnancy. It also has a Yin aspect in that it also nourishes the fetus and the maturation of the eggs in the follicles.

Normal menstruation and fertility depend mainly on the state of Kidney Essence, Heart Qi and Heart Blood. Deficiencies of one of these can lead to the absence of periods and infertility.

The health of the Uterus is also related to the proper functioning of the Liver and Spleen. Normal functioning of these organs ensures a proper material basis for conception.

Yin and Yang

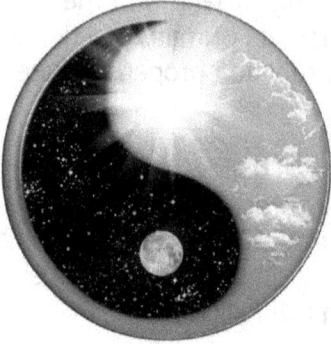

In order to better comprehend the functioning of Traditional Chinese Medicine it is useful to understand the concept of Yin and Yang.

Qi or life energy is made up of two complimentary and opposing forces called Yin and Yang. Yin and Yang are two sides of the same Qi coin. One cannot exist without the other. Yin is dark, passive and feminine. Yang is light, active, and masculine. All things are made of both Yin and Yang that naturally balance each other.

The Moon is Yin. The Sun is Yang. Yin conserves, contracts and descends. Yang transforms, expands and rises. Yin is inside and restful. Yang is outside and active. Yin is opposite to Yang. They are two stages of a cyclical movement one constantly changing into the other, such as day turning into night, summer into winter, and growth into decay.

If this waxing and waning exceeds the bodies normal energetic limits and loses its dynamic equilibrium, deficient or excess Yin or Yang will occur, leading to the development of abnormalities and illness.

The first half of the menstrual cycle is governed by Yin energy reflecting the predominance of estrogen which moistens the Uterus and thickens the endometrial lining in preparation for ovulation. The increasing Yin also supports the production of Blood and produces sperm friendly mucus during ovulation.

The second half of the menstrual cycle is governed by Yang energy and the production of progesterone secreted after ovulation by the corpus luteum, which heats up the Uterus, transforms the endometrial lining so it can hold a fertilized ovum, and allows for the descending movement of ovulation.

Energy Anatomy

Western medicine looks at the reproductive system from the point of view of the physical body and its various physiological processes. Traditional Chinese Medicine sees the same system but through the eyes of the energy body.

For a TCM practitioner it is important to understand the energy systems that are involved in the reproductive function. This helps develop more targeted treatment protocols that will increase the chances of fertility both in men and women.

The reproductive organs are in the lower abdomen called the Lower Dantian. In TCM the Lower Dantian is called the Lower Jiao or Triple Burner. The extraordinary meridians involved in reproduction are the Bao Mai or Uterus Vessel, Ren Mai or Conception Vessel, Du Mai or Governing Vessel, Chong Mai or Penetrating Vessel, and the Dai Mai or Girdling Vessel. The Bao Mai or Uterus Vessel originates in the Heart and connects with the Uterus.

An acupuncture point, located in the depression under the spinous process of the 2nd lumbar vertebra called the Ming Men, Gate of Fire or Gate of Life, is also an important point when treating issues related to conception.

The major organ systems involved in conception are the Kidneys, Heart, Liver and Spleen. The major ordinary meridians are the Liver and Kidney Meridians.

Lower Dantian

The Lower Dantian or House of the Earthly Realm contains the Uterus in Women and the Room of Sperm in Men. It is primarily responsible for physical strength, sexual vitality and overall health.

The Kidneys reside in the Lower Dantian. Kidney Essence or Jing is the origin of sperm in men and menstrual Blood and ova in women.

Yuan Qi (Original or Ancestral Qi) originates in the Ming Men and resides in the Lower Dantian. Yuan Qi is sometimes called Jing or Essence in Motion.

Uterus Vessel - Place of the Child

The Heart is closely connected to the Uterus through the Uterus Vessel or Bao Mai explaining the profound influence on the Uterus of mental-emotional problems affecting the Heart. The Kidneys are also closely connected to the Uterus via the Bao Luo or Uterus Channel.

A normal menstruation, ovulation, and sexual function in women and the sexual function in men rely in part on the coordination and harmony of the Kidneys and the Heart. The Water of the Kidneys and the Fire of the Heart must nourish and balance each other.

The Heart is connected to the Kidneys:
- Within the Chong Mai, Uterus Vessel and Shao Yin Channels,
- Indirectly via the Du Mai and Ren Mai, both of which flow through the Heart and originate from the space between the Kidneys.

The discharge of Blood at menstruation and the release of the eggs at ovulation depend on the descending of Heart Qi. When the period does not come it means the Uterus Vessel is obstructed.

Coordination between the descending of Heart Fire and ascending of Kidney Water ensures a normal menstruation and ovulation in women and normal sexual function in both men and women. Both the Du and Ren Mai also have a profound influence on sexuality and sexual function including sexual desire, sexual arousal, erection, maintenance of erection, and ejaculation.

Uterus Vessel issues can be treated by activating the Chong Mai. In men we can use the Heart channel points to treat sexual dysfunctions such as impotence or premature ejaculation which are often due to Heart Qi not descending to the Lower Burner to communicate and link with the Kidneys.

Extraordinary Vessels - Ren, Du & Chong Mai

The Ren, Du and Chong Mai govern embryological development and control the energies that determine growth, maturation and aging. These three meridians represent the Hypothalamic-Pituitary-Ovarian Access (HPO)

They originate in the space between the Kidneys and flow through the Uterus. The menstrual function depends on the proper functioning of the Ren, Du and Chong Vessels. Du represents Yang, Ren represents Yin, and Chong represents Blood.

Ren Mai

The Ren Mai, the Sea of Yin, Essence and Fluids, is closely related to all problems of the reproductive system including the internal and external genitalia in women. It is used in TCM to remove obstructions to the movement Qi and Blood, facilitating conception, fertility and pregnancy.

The Ren Mai develops the ovaries, nourishes Yin after menopause and reduces the effects of Empty Heat from Yin deficiency. The Ren Mai starts at the Ming Men or Gate of Life, running down to Ren 1, located at the center of the pelvic floor, travelling up the anterior midline of the body to the mouth, circling the mouth before entering the eyes at ST 1.

Du Mai

The Du Mai is the Sea of Yang and Qi. It develops the medulla and the cerebellum. Its primary function is the Yang aspect of a person's health. It directly affects the Gate of Life and along with the Ren Vessel, influences the hormonal aspect of the menstrual cycle (Hypothalamus-Pituitary-Ovarian Axis).

The path of the Du Mai starts at the Gates of Vitality, running down to Ren 1 before moving to Du 1 located between the tip of the coccyx and the anus. It then ascends the midline up the spine entering the brain and skull, ending at DU 28 in the upper lip.

The Du Mai also goes to the front of the body to the genitals and penis in men and to the vagina and vulva in women. It has an abdominal branch which follows the path of the Ren Mai to the Heart, throat, chin and eyes.

Du and Ren Mai

The Du and Ren vessels represent the HPO axis responsible for ovulation. In the fluctuation of Yin and Yang during the menstrual cycle:
- The Du Mai and Ren Mai form a closed circuit and may be looked

upon as one channel called the Micro Cosmic Orbit
- The Du Mai represents the Kidney Yang (Progesterone)
- The Ren Mai represents the Kidney Yin (Estrogen)
- Their proper functioning is essential to fertility

Chong Mai

The Chong Mai or Sea of Blood provides the foundation of Du and Ren. The Chong Mai influences the supply and proper movement of Blood in the Uterus and controls the hormonal cycle as well as all aspects of menstruation. Its primary function is to move and regulate Qi and Blood. It also develops the adrenals and their cortex.

The Chong Mai starts at the Gates of Vitality, runs to Ren 1 where it meets the Du and Ren meridians, emerges at ST 30, located on the lower abdomen level with the superior border of the pubic symphysis, and continues up the Kidney channel to Kid 21, located on the upper abdomen, and then internally to the Heart, chin, mouth and forehead.

From ST 30 it also moves down the legs to meet the Kidney and Spleen Channels. Therefore, the powerful Qi of the Chong Mai moves simultaneously in two directions, up the body and down the legs. Liv 3 and SP 6 strongly activate the energy of the Chong Mai.

The Chong Mai influences the whole body as it is connected to most major organ systems. Changes in the Uterus may affect the Stomach via the Chong Mai. The Chong Mai nourishes skin with Blood and allows for the growth of body hair. Menstruation depletes Blood therefore women do not grow facial hair. The Chong Mai also controls the Zong muscles in the abdomen which many be interpreted as being the penis.

Blood Stasis of the Chong Mai is also considered as Liver Blood Stasis. This pathology is treated through the Liver. Rebellious Qi of the Chong Mai manifests mostly through the Liver Meridian.

Deficiencies of the Chong Mai are mainly related to the Kidneys, and occasionally to the Spleen and the Heart. Blood Stasis or Stagnation of Qi in the Chong Mai may cause painful periods. Absence of Blood may lead to an absence of periods.

The functions of the Chong and Ren Mai overlap. Ren Mai nourishes Kidney Yin. The Chong Mai has domain over Blood. The Ren Mai is used to treat irregular, absent and late periods. The Chong Mai is used to treat PMS, painful periods, heavy periods, irregular periods, Blood Stasis, accumulation of Phlegm and Endometriosis.

Hormonal changes driven by the actions of the Ren, Du and Chong Mai can deregulate the menstrual cycle. When the Ren Mai becomes deficient and the Chong Mai is depleted, the Tian Gui dries up, signaling the arrival of menopause in women.

Dai Mai - Belt Cannel

The Dai Mai or Belt Channel surrounds the body at the hips facilitating balance and the vertical movement of Qi. The Dai Mai cannot be too tight or too loose to allow the descending of Kidney Qi, the rising of Spleen Qi, and the smooth flow of Liver Qi.

The Dai Mai guides and supports the Qi of the Uterus and the Kidney Essence. It encircles the waist passing through GB 26, GB 27, GB 28, Liv 13 and BL 23.

The main pathologies in gynecology treated by the Dai Mai involve Dampness, normally from Spleen Qi Deficiency, infusing downwards causing excessive vaginal discharge. The Dai Mai is also involved in preventing miscarriages by stabilizing the fetus, and in treating prolapse of the Uterus, dampness in the genital region, blocked fallopian tubes, ovarian cysts and abdominal pain from painful periods.

Ming Men or Gate of Life

The Minister Fire of the Gate of Life represents the physiological Fire within the Kidneys. It is the root of the Yuan or Original Qi from which the Du, Ren and Chong Mai originate.

The Fire warms the Uterus and balances the influence of Yin. A Deficiency of Minister Fire indicates a weakness of Kidney Yang. Since the Minister Fire nourishes Water there may also be secondary Kidney Yin Deficiency.

The Minister Fire promotes the transformation of Kidney Jing into Tian Gui, which turns into menstrual Blood. The Minister Fire makes conception possible by enabling the maturation of the follicles and the production of ova.

The Minister Fire from the Kidneys is without form and generates Water, which builds Essence. The Fire and Water within the Kidneys are inseparable and interdependent. In contrast, the Emperor Fire of the Heart has form and overcomes Water.

If the Minister Fire is deficient and does not warm the Uterus, it can lead to accumulation of Cold obstructing the Uterus, painful periods and infertility as well as a lack of sexual desire. If the Minister Fire is excessive, it heats the Blood causing excessive menstrual bleeding, infertility or miscarriage.

The Minister Fire also warms and nourishes the Room of Sperm. When it is deficient, the Room of Sperm is cold, and this may cause impotence or lack of libido. When it is excessive, it flares upwards affecting the Heart and Pericardium.

During sexual excitation the Minister Fire within the Kidneys is aroused and flows up towards the Pericardium and Heart. For this reason, the person becomes flushed in the face as the complexion is a manifestation of the Heart, and the Heart rate increases.

With orgasm and ejaculation, there is a downward movement of Qi which releases the accumulated Minister Fire downwards. For this to occur normally the downward movement of Heart Qi is crucial.

If the Minister Fire within the Kidneys is deficient there will be a decreased libido in both men and women, an inability to reach an orgasm in women, and impotence in men. If Heart Qi and Heart Blood are deficient or not descending to communicate with the Kidneys, there may be impotence or premature ejaculation in men and an inability to reach an orgasm in women even in the presence of sexual arousal.

In summary, a normal sexual desire, arousal, erection and orgasm therefore relies on three main factors:

- The ascending of Kidney Water and descending of Heart Fire
- The communication between Kidneys and Heart. Heart Qi and Heart Blood need to flow downwards to the Lower Burner to interact with Blood and Jing.
- The connection between Du and Ren Mai.

Kidneys

The Kidneys are the main organ system involved in fertility. They are the origin of Tian Gui or Menstrual Blood, and store Jing or Essence, the generic material received from our parents.

The Kidneys govern growth and development. They are responsible for bone and teeth formation, overall brain function and control water balance and elimination.

Kidney Yin and Kidney Yang are the foundation of the Yin and Yang of the whole body. Kidney Yin and Yang rely on each other for their existence. Kidney Yin provides the material basis for Kidney Yang. Kidney Yang provides the necessary heat for all Kidney functions. The movement of Yin to Yang, and Yang to Yin during the menstrual cycle reflects the movement of Kidney Yin and Kidney Yang.

Kidney Jing governs the process of human reproduction and development. Strong Jing is essential in promoting fertility. The Minister Fire is the Yang aspect of Jing while the Yin aspect is the Jing itself that at puberty crystalizes into Menstrual Blood and ova.

When the Jing is abundant, the constitution is strong, the women is fertile, and the fetus develops normally. When the Jing is deficient, the constitution is weak, the women is often infertile, and the fetus may not develop normally.

Kidney Jing nourishes the Uterus and thickens the uterine lining. The Kidneys determine when women menstruate and when they go into menopause. Because the Kidneys reside in the lower back, menstrual problems accompanied by lower back pain often involve the Kidneys.

Most infertility cases characterised by a deficiency of Jing manifest as an ovulatory dysfunction as ovulation is an expression of the transformation of Kidney Jing into ova. Therefore, to promote ovulation one must nourish Jing.

In a normal monthly cycle, the release of Follicle Stimulating Hormones (FSH) stimulates the women's ovaries to produce estrogen and begin follicular development. Reinforcing the Kidneys in women with healthy ovaries can stimulate them to respond normally to FSH and help produce higher levels of estrogen favoring the development of healthy follicles and eggs. In women suffering from Premature Ovarian Failure reinforcing the Kidneys can help restore normal levels of FSH.

Heart

The Heart communicates with the Kidneys in promoting a healthy sexuality, ovulation and menstruation. During the menstrual cycle, it plays an important role in the transformation of Yin to Yang at ovulation, and Yang to Yin at the start of the period.

The descending of Heart Qi to the Uterus promotes the descending of menstrual Blood during the menses, and of the ovum at ovulation. Heart Yang aids the Kidney Essence form Tian Gui or Menstrual Blood.

The Heart governs the Blood and has a similar influence on the menstrual cycle as Liver Blood. Heart Blood Deficiency can lead to scanty periods, Heart Blood Stasis can lead to painful periods, and Heart Blood Heat can lead to heavy periods.

Liver

The Liver is connected to the Chong Mai or Penetrating Vessel. Its prime responsibility is to move Qi and Blood, which represent the Yang and Yin aspects of the Liver.

There is a direct connection between Liver Blood and Tian Gui or Menstrual Blood. The two influence each other. The Blood stored in the Uterus is a combination of Tian Gui from the Kidneys, and post-natal Blood from the Qi of the Stomach and Spleen.

The Liver is involved in all transformations in the body, including ovulation. It regulates, stores and filters Blood and metabolises hormones.

In the pre-menstrual phase of the menstrual cycle the Liver moves the Blood from other parts of the body to the Uterus in preparation of the menses. During this phase Liver Blood Deficiency can lead to the absence of periods, scanty or late periods.

Emotional stress makes the Liver lose its ability to smooth emotional energy which can impede its transformation functions affecting ovulation and menstruation.

Liver Qi Stagnation causes hormones like estrogen to build up in the body contributing to endometriosis, PCOS, and cancer. A Liver imbalance can confine the Qi to a small space creating heat which ascends the Gall Bladder meridian causing premenstrual migraines.

Spleen

The Spleen governs digestion and elimination. Together with the Stomach, the Spleen is the source of acquired Qi and Blood. It also holds the Blood in place both in the vessels and in the Uterus helping to prevent excessive bleeding during menses as well as prolapse of the Uterus.

The Spleen is often implicated in bleeding disorders as well as in many instances of Luteal Phase Defect in which spotting precedes menstruation. During menstruation Spleen Qi Deficiency will manifest as low energy levels and loose stools with heavy bleeding and thin, watery Blood which is almost pink in color.

Lungs

The Lungs exercise a minor influence on the menstrual function. The Lungs govern the Qi. Qi Deficiency of the Lungs and Spleen can lead to prolapse of the Uterus and heavy periods. Sadness and grief deplete Lung Qi which can lead to stoppage of the menses.

Liver & Kidney Channels

The genitals are related primarily to the Liver and Kidney channels, and to the Ren, Chong and Du Mai. The Liver Main, Luo, Divergent and Muscle channels wrap around the genitalia. The Kidney Main, Luo and Muscle channels flow through the genitalia.

The influence of the Ren Mai on the genitalia is obvious. The influence of the Du Mai Vessel is often overlooked. Ancient Chinese medical texts describe an anterior branch of the Du Mai Vessel that flows to the external genitalia both in men and women, and to the pubic bone and from here ascends the abdomen on the same trajectory as the Ren Mai. The branch of the Du Mai going to the penis in men and vagina in women has clinical significance because it means that the Du Mai rather than the Ren Mai can be used for genital problems in both men and women when there is a pronounced Kidney Yang deficiency.

Patterns of Disharmony

Major patterns of disharmony related to infertility:

- Deficiency of Kidney Qi, Yang, Yin or Jing
- Blood Stasis
- Blood Deficiency
- Liver Qi Stagnation
- Heart and Kidney Not Communicating
- Cold in the Uterus
- Accumulation of Phlegm and Dampness

When diagnosing infertility in women first identify whether you are dealing primarily with an Excess or a Deficient condition. With Deficient conditions, infertility is due to a lack of vital substances essential for conception such as Blood or Jing. The two main Deficiencies are Kidney Deficiency (Qi, Yin & Yang), or Blood Deficiency.

Kidney Jing is always a factor in both its Yin and Yang aspects, which must be perfectly balanced for fertilization to occur. The production and fertilisation of the egg depends on strong Yin. The Minister Fire of the Ming Men provides the spark to activate the Yin Water enabling it to fertilize and nourish the egg.

The Yin and Yang aspects of Jing provide the foundation for conception by producing the eggs while the Minister Fire plays an essential role in transforming the eggs into a foetus.

With Full conditions, fertilisation cannot occur because the Uterus, Ren and Chong Vessels are obstructed by pathogenic factors such as Cold, Blood Heat, Damp Phlegm or Blood Stasis.

Kidney Qi Deficiency

The Kidneys are the source of all reproductive and sexual functions. Weak Kidneys affect the quality of a man's sperm and the quality and development of a women's eggs and Uterus.

The Kidneys exercise the strongest influence on the Uterus. In some cases, weak Kidney Qi can cause delayed periods, cessation of menstruation and infertility. Weak Kidney Qi can hamper IVF treatments by reducing the amount and quality of harvested eggs. In men, weak Kidneys can cause erectile dysfunction.

S/S of Kidney Qi Deficiency

Lack of energy, lower back pain, lower libido or sex drive, weak ejaculation, pain in knee or ankle area, frequent urination, especially at night when sleeping, and irregular periods.

S/S Kidney Yin Deficiency

Dizziness, tinnitus, vertigo, sore back, constipation, empty heat signs such as flushed face, night sweats, hot palms, feet and chest, hot flashes, leucorrhea, and chronic dry throat. Related conditions are insomnia, menopausal syndrome, and various anxiety disorders, menstrual irregularities, as well as genital and reproductive problems related to heat and dryness.

S/S Kidney Yang Deficiency

Sore or weak back and knees, sensation of cold, aversion to cold, weak lower limbs, fatigue, clear copious urine, poor appetite, loose stools, impotence and edema. Related conditions are chronic fatigue syndrome, chronic back pain, and infertility. Cold sperm and eggs are infertile as cold reduces sperm count and delays or blocks egg release.

S/S Kidney Jing Deficiency

Kidney Jing Deficiency includes symptoms of Kidney Qi, Yin and Yang Deficiency. It is differentiated primarily by the absence of symptoms of Heat or Cold. In addition, look for:

- Premature degeneration of bones and teeth
- Premature aging
- Infertility: reduced sperm count or weak eggs
- Delayed or absent menses
- Deficiency of semen or vaginal fluids
- Loss of sexual desire or energy
- Sluggish physical movements
- Impaired mental functions

Blood Stasis

Blood Stasis is a major pathology affecting fertility in women. It involves mainly the Liver Organ system and the Chong Mai. When treating complicated cases of infertility always suspect Blood Stasis.

Blood Stasis can lead over time to uterine fibroids, carcinoma, tumors, strokes, coronary heart disease, endometriosis, cancer and fibroids of the breasts, abdominal masses, infertility, and painful periods.

Blood Stasis in women derives mainly from Qi Stagnation and external Cold invading the Uterus. The presence of Phlegm can be an aggravating factor. Other contributing factors can be damage to the Uterus during a previous delivery and long-term illness.

Blood Stasis impairs the proper functioning of the Ren and Chong Mai. A woman's menstruation can become irregular and conception may be difficult. Women suffering from Blood Stasis can present with a normal tongue. In more advanced cases the tongue becomes purple. Dark menstrual Blood with clots remains the major indicator of the presence of Blood Stasis in gynecological conditions.

Blood Stasis may lead to additional patterns of disharmony such as Blood Deficiency. In addition, although excessive bleeding is normally caused by Spleen Qi Deficiency or Blood Heat, Blood Stasis may aggravate the condition.

Blood Deficiency

Women are very prone to Blood Deficiency partly from the monthly loss of Blood occurring with the periods, and partly from diet, overwork, and emotional stress.

Blood Deficiency has many different manifestations and is often the root of many other patterns. Blood Deficiency in most cases means Liver Blood Deficiency because the Liver houses Blood. However, the Heart governs Blood and Heart Blood Deficiency is also common.

Also, the Spleen makes Gu Qi which is the origin of Blood and so a deficiency of the Spleen may also lead to Blood Deficiency. In addition, the Kidneys store Jing Qi. Jing Qi produces marrow which generates bone marrow which contributes to making Blood.

Also, if the patient has weak Yuan or Jing Qi, the body will have difficulty making Blood as the Yuan and Jing Qi facilitate the process.

Clinical manifestations of Blood Deficiency include pale or sallow complexion, pale lips, dizziness, poor memory, dry eyes, blurring of vision, poor night vision, palpitations, insomnia, numbness of the hands and feet, absent or scanty menstruation, a pale tongue and thready pulse.

Liver Qi Stagnation

The Liver stores Blood and moves Qi and Blood. It provides Blood to the Uterus in close co-ordination with the Chong Mai. Emotional and reproductive health depend on a smooth flow of Qi and Blood. In cases of emotional disturbances, especially frustration and anger, the Liver's regulating functions are impaired resulting in stagnation of Liver Qi.

When internal Qi and Blood flow become disharmonious, the extra meridians are affected, and the menses will not come regularly hindering conception.

Clinical manifestations include irritability, tendency to anger, dizziness, abdominal and hypochondriac pain and distension, fullness in the chest, excessive sighing, breast distension, belching, loss of appetite, nausea, sensation of a foreign body in the throat, menstrual disorders, and a wiry pulse.

Liver Qi Stagnation is often accompanied by elevated levels of certain hormones such as prolactin and estrogen. Resolving Liver Qi Stagnation helps the body metabolize these excess hormones.

Heart / Uterus Connection

The Heart is closely connected with the Uterus through the Uterus Vessel. This explains the profound influence on the Uterus of mental-emotional problems affecting the Heart.

There is also another important connection and that is via Blood. The Heart provides Blood to the Uterus. The Heart governs Blood and the Uterus stores Blood. Although most gynecologists will emphasize the role of Liver Blood in relation to the Uterus, some put the accent on

Heart Blood. According to this approach, tonifying the Heart will help Kidney Jing or Essential Energy produce menstrual Blood.

Normal menstruation and fertility depend on the state of the Kidney Essence and Heart Blood. If Heart Blood is deficient Heart Qi does not descend to the Uterus. If the Kidney Essence is deficient, menstruation does not occur. A deficiency in either Heart or Kidneys can therefore cause infertility or amenorrhea.

In general deficiencies of Heart Qi and Heart Yang involve more physical symptoms. They move the Blood and provide the active function of circulation. Heart Qi and Heart Yang are closely related, Heart Yang being a broader, more inclusive category.

Deficiency of Heart Blood and Yin involve more mental-emotional disturbances, and somewhat fewer physical symptoms. Blood and Yin house the mental consciousness. Emotional upsets may influence the uteruses' ability to nourish a developing fetus. When disorders of the Uterus and Heart arise treat the Penetrating Vessel.

Cold in the Uterus

Cold in the Uterus is a frequent cause of infertility. For conception to occur, the temperature of the Uterus should be even and warm, not too hot nor too cold.

Cold obstructs the Uterus, Ren and Chong Vessels, which can lead to Blood Stasis. It also dampens the Ming Men Fire hindering fertilization. Cold causes the Blood to congeal and become sluggish. This leads to pain and Cold in the lower abdomen made better by Heat, and other symptoms such as cold limbs, painful menstrual periods, delayed menstruation with dark purple clots, a pale tongue, and a pulse that feels deep and slow.

Cold in the Uterus can be a Full or Empty condition depending on the level of Kidney Yang Deficiency. The pulse is an important factor in distinguishing Empty (Weak overall. May be slightly tight on the left pulse rear position) from Full Cold (Full & Tight).

When Liver Blood is deficient the Uterus is empty and vulnerable, so it can be easily invaded by Cold. When Cold obstructs the Uterus, Liver

Blood cannot be stored properly, and this may lead to Blood Deficiency. Thus, Liver Blood Deficiency and Cold often coexist.

To diagnosis a Cold Uterus, use the back of the hand to compare the temperature of the lower abdomen to the area above the navel and to the forehead. Sometimes the cold in the lower abdomen will only manifest during menses.

Accumulation of Dampness & Phlegm

Damp phlegm invades the body from the Lower Burner preventing the proper movement of Qi and Blood, which can lead to stagnation of Qi and Blood Stasis. The meridians around the Uterus (Ren & Chong) are obstructed and unable to gather Jing resulting in irregular menses and conception problems.

Improper dietary habits or Yang Deficiency in the Kidneys and Spleen lead to dysfunction in the water metabolism and cause Phlegm and Dampness to accumulate, disrupting the movement of Qi and Blood.

Accumulation of Dampness and Phlegm combined with Blood Stasis can lead over time to the formation of ovarian cysts, uterine fibroids or polyps.

Summary

The Uterus, Ren and Chong Vessels are always involved in both Full and Empty conditions affecting fertility. In Deficiency cases the Uterus, Ren and Chong Mai lack the necessary nourishment to nurture the fertilized egg. In Excess cases, pathogenic factors obstruct these structures preventing the proper transformation of Qi, Blood and Jing.

Balance Energy/Improve Blood Flow

Blood delivers nutrients, hormones, and oxygen throughout the body. For women who are trying to conceive, Blood helps nourish and balance the reproductive organs. Improved Blood flow is essential to support the reproductive organs in their task of conception.

Qi and Blood work hand in hand. Blood is a denser form of Qi. Qi gives life and movement to Blood, whereas Blood nourishes the organs that produce the Qi. Like Yin and Yang, one cannot exist without the other.

TCM treatments for infertility focus on building and balancing the flow of Qi, and enhancing Blood flow which helps:

- Facilitate natural pregnancy by regulating the menstrual cycle and balancing hormonal levels
- Reduce the stress of infertility and its related treatments by releasing endorphins in the brain
- Improve ovary or testicle health resulting in better egg or sperm quality
- Improve ovarian function and provide a thick, rich uterine lining
- Alleviate menstrual issues such as PMS and breast distension
- Reduce the risk of miscarriage and ectopic pregnancy
- Reduce common symptoms like morning sickness, nausea, and aches and pains (low back pain, for example)
- Increase the success rates of IVF and IUI
- Promote a healthy diet and lifestyle

TCM can treat all common disorders related to infertility such as:

- Anxiety
- Irregular Menstruation Cycle
- Endometriosis
- Cold Uterus
- Ovarian Cysts including Polycystic Ovary Syndrome (PCOS)
- Uterine Fibroids
- Ovulation issues
- Pelvic Inflammatory Disease
- Luteal Phase Defect

To achieve better treatment results, acupuncture is often combined with Chinese herbal formulas. In women under 39 years old, with the acupuncture/herbal combo it may take from 6 to 12 months to restore fertility. Patients also feel healthier due to their balanced physiological and emotional state.

Acupuncture and herbs will not address tubal adhesions which can occur because of Pelvic Inflammatory Disease or Endometriosis. Nevertheless, a person can still benefit from improved ovarian and follicular function.

Acupuncture is generally safe as a treatment for infertility regardless of a person's medical history. Although the risk of miscarriage may increase if counter-indicated points are used during pregnancy.

Discussion on Blood

The Discussion on Blood written in 1884 by Tang Zong Hai says: "Fire is Yang and generates Blood which is Yin. On the other hand, Blood nourishes Fire and makes sure Fire does not flare up, whilst Blood moistens the lower Burner. It is stored in the Liver, it fills the Sea of Blood and the Chong, Ren and Dai Mai, and it warms and nourishes the whole body."

"When Blood moistens the Lower Burner and the Sea of Blood, and Heart Fire follows it down to the umbilicus, then Blood is flourishing, and Fire does not flare excessively, so that men are free of disease and women are fertile."

Menstrual Blood - Tian Gui

The famous Qing dynasty gynecologist Fu Qing Zhu (1607-1684) stressed that menstrual Blood is not Blood but Water or Tian Gui, which originates in the Kidneys. Tian Gui is formed from Kidney Yin but with the participation of Heart Yang. Despite being Blood-Red in color, it is not Blood, hence its name Tian Gui.

According to the internationally renowned author, Giovanni Maciocia, in women, there are two types of Blood:

- Ordinary Blood stored by the Liver that nourishes hair, sinews, nails and eyes and houses the Hun (Cloud or Ethereal Soul) and
- Menstrual Blood that is Tian Gui

There is a connection between these two types of Blood and that connection takes place through the Liver. Therefore, a woman who suffers from scanty periods from a deficiency of Tian Gui may also have symptoms and signs of Blood Deficiency such as dry hair or blurred vision.

Tain Gui is associated with the development of the male and female reproductive function and the natural ability to give birth to offspring. Tian Gui is also used to describe seminal and menstrual fluids.

Tian means heaven with two aspects:
- Pre-heaven
- Post-heaven

That which is given at birth is pre-heaven. It includes not only ancestral and hereditary factors, DNA, and genes, but also astrological and karmic influences.

That which comes after birth is post-heaven. This is nourishment, food and water, the air we breathe, and the physical and emotional environments we live in.

The pre-heaven and post-heaven are mutually dependent. The pre-heaven offers potentials and sets limits; the post-heaven enables the expression of these potentials. The pre-heaven is the seed; the post-heaven is the soil, the water, and the sun.

Maciocia adds that Tian Gui is not just menstrual Blood but encompasses the ova from the ovaries, the mature female reproductive cells. "When Tian Gui arrives a girl can conceive, but it is the follicles in the ovaries, and not menstrual Blood, that renders her fertile."

In the classic text on Chinese Medicine, Su Wen, Shang Gu Tian Zhen Lun Pian states: "In females at the age of seven the Kidney Qi is in fullness, the teeth change and the hair grows, at two times seven the Tian Gui matures, the conception vessel is open, the Sea of Blood Vessel Chong Mai is full and the monthly affair flows down in a timely manner, hence she can have children. "

"In males at the age of eight the Kidney Qi is in repletion (Full), the hair grows and the teeth change, (Second teeth grow), at two times eight the Kidney is abundant, the Tian Gui has arrived, the Essence Qi overflows, (when) the Yin and Yang unite, children can be conceived....."

This clearly illustrates that both male and female have Tian Gui and that it influences the human growth, development and production of a type of Essence in the reproductive organs.

The fact that the menstrual cycle starts at 14 indicates that the ovaries already have developed their normal physiological function and that ovulation is taking place. In the male at age 16, the Kidney Qi is sufficient to create spermatic fluid, so if male and female have sexual intercourse, pregnancy may ensue.

In women after the age of 49 the sexual functions have declined, menstruation stops, procreation has ceased, the breasts, Uterus and vagina gradually shrink and withdraw from the beginning of menopause until full cessation of menstruation.

In men at age 56 the Liver Qi declines, the tendons and ligaments become stiff, the sperm is reduced, the Kidney Qi weakens, the body has reached its limit... indicating a gradual decline of the reproductive system.

Growth, development and aging rely to a large degree on the regulatory function of the endocrine system, such as the anterior lobe of the pituitary gland, which secrets gonadotropic hormone, thyroid stimulating hormones, human growth hormones and prolactin etc.

Tian Gui mirrors the normal physiological stages of hormonal development. If the hypothalamic and pituitary secretions are normal, then the human growth and development remain normal.

Tian Gui is intimately related to the abundance or weakness of the Kidney Qi. If the Kidney Qi is abundant, then the Tian Gui or sexual capacity and fertility are strong. If the Kidney Qi is weak, the Tian Gui or sexual capacity and fertility are weak.

Menstruation Facts

According to Western medical theory, the average age for a girl to get her first period is 12, but the age range is about eight to 15 years old. Most of the time, the first period starts about two years after breasts first start to develop. If a girl has not had her first period by age 15, or if it has been more than two to three years since breast growth started with no periods, she should see a doctor.

Women usually have periods until menopause. Menopause occurs between the ages of 45 and 55, usually around age 50. Menopause means that a woman is no longer ovulating or having periods and can no longer get pregnant.

The time when the body begins its move into menopause is called the menopausal transition which can last anywhere from two to eight years. Some women have early menopause because of surgery or other treatment, illness, or other reasons.

If women don't have a period for 90 days, they should see a doctor to check for pregnancy, early menopause, or other health problems that can cause periods to stop or become irregular.

The menstrual cycle is a recurring cycle in which the endometrial lining of the Uterus prepares for pregnancy. If pregnancy does not occur the lining, which contains Blood and tissue, is shed at menstruation through the cervix and vagina.

A cycle is counted from the first full day of the period to the first day of the next period. The average menstrual cycle is 28 days and can range anywhere from 26 to 32 days in adults and from 21 to 45 days in young teens.

The regularity of the cycle is very important. If the length of a cycle varies from month to month within what is considered as being a normal range, it would still be considered an abnormal cycle.

A regular menstrual cycle is a sign that important parts of the reproductive system are working normally. The menstrual cycle is a hormonal driven cycle. During the month the rise and fall of levels of hormones, mainly estrogen and progesterone, control the menstrual cycle and prepare the body for pregnancy.

In the first half of the cycle, levels of estrogen start to rise. Estrogen plays an important role in keeping the patient healthy, especially by helping build strong bones and keeping them strong over time. Estrogen also makes the lining of the Uterus grow and thicken.

The lining of the Uterus will nourish the embryo if a pregnancy occurs. While the lining of the Uterus is growing, an egg or ovum starts to mature in one of the ovaries. At about day 14 of an average 28-day cycle, the egg leaves the ovary. After the egg has left the ovary, it travels through the fallopian tube to the Uterus. Hormone levels rise and help prepare the uterine lining for pregnancy.

A woman becomes pregnant if the egg is fertilized by a man's sperm and attaches to the uterine wall. If the egg is not fertilized, it will break apart, the hormone levels drop, and the thickened lining of the Uterus is shed during the menstrual period.

Most periods vary somewhat. The flow may be light, moderate or heavy and can vary in length. With age, the cycle usually shortens and becomes more regular. Problems with periods include amenorrhea (no period), dysmenorrhea (painful period), abnormal bleeding and Blood clots.

According to TCM the menstrual cycle is driven by the ebb and flow of the Kidney Yin (estrogen) and Kidney Yang (progesterone). At the start of the menses, Yin starts to increase reaching its maximum at mid-cycle around ovulation at which point it starts to decrease. Yang increases at mid-cycle rising rapidly in the days before the period, decreasing at the start of the period.

There is a switch from Yang to Yin at the start of the period and from Yin to Yang at mid-cycle around ovulation. The change from Yin to Yang and Yang to Yin is initiated in part by Heart Qi and Heart Blood and is marked by the discharge of Blood as well as by the discharge of the ovum or ova.

Day 1 starts with the first day of the period. This occurs after hormone levels drop at the end of the previous cycle, signaling Blood and tissues lining the Uterus to break down and shed from the body. Bleeding lasts about 5 days.

Usually by **Day 7**, bleeding has stopped. Leading up to this time, hormones cause fluid-filled pockets called follicles to develop on the ovaries. Each follicle contains an egg.

Between **Day 7 and 14**, one follicle will continue to develop and reach maturity. The lining of the Uterus starts to thicken, waiting for the implantation of a fertilized egg. The lining is rich in Blood and nutrients.

Around **Day 14** (in a 28-day cycle), hormones cause the mature follicle to burst and release an egg from the ovary, a process called ovulation.

Over the next few days, the egg travels down the fallopian tube towards the Uterus. If a sperm unites with the egg here, the fertilized egg will continue down the fallopian tube and attach to the lining of the Uterus.

If the egg is not fertilized, hormone levels will drop around **Day 25**. This signals the next menstrual cycle to begin. The egg will break apart and be shed with the next period.

An Egg Takes a Long Time to Mature

Most eggs are present within the ovary in an immature state from the time of a woman's first menstruation. Some eggs will lie dormant for years or even decades before they begin to mature, while others will degenerate and never develop.

For eggs to complete their journey to ovulation, they receive a signal to begin their final maturation process about 150 days before they would be released from the ovary.

At the beginning of any given cycle, there are generally about 12 eggs that have started to grow and as ovulation nears, preference is given to one of those eggs, as it receives the final push to maturity and is then released from the ovary.

Once the egg has matured and is released from the ovary during ovulation, it goes into the fallopian tube where it lives for 12 to 24 hours.

The Egg Has a Short Life After Ovulation

Conception is possible if sperm is already present in the fallopian tubes when the egg is released, or if a woman has sex while the egg is alive, causing sperm to swim up through the Uterus into the fallopian tube.

Sperm can reach the egg in as little as 30 minutes. If conception is successful, the newly fertilized egg will travel out of the fallopian tube and implant into the Uterus six to 10 days later. If the egg is not fertilized, it will simply dissolve and pass out with the menstrual flow.

Though the egg has a lifespan of less than a day, sperm can stay alive inside a woman's Uterus and fallopian tubes anywhere from 1 to 5 days. Sex up to 5 days prior to ovulation can result in pregnancy! The lifespan of the sperm is dependent on the sperm's health, but also on the woman's cervical fluid, which can nourish the sperm during its wait.

Pinpointing Fertile Time

When it comes to conception, timing is everything. Once ovulation occurs – the moment at which the egg is released from the ovary and pushed down the fallopian tube – the clock starts ticking. An egg is only viable for up to 24 hours after ovulation, so sperm must get to work immediately if fertilization is going to be successful.

For the very best chance of conceiving, sperm must be ready and waiting in the fallopian tube when the egg is released. But, because sperm can only live for 3 to 5 days inside the female reproductive tract, there are only a few days during each menstrual cycle during which intercourse can lead to conception. Therefore, predicting ovulation is essential when trying to conceive.

A variety of ways are used to identify the fertile window. Some women can pinpoint their fertile days by watching for changes in the consistency of their cervical mucus (the presence of "egg-white" cervical mucus can indicate that ovulation is just around the corner), or by charting their basal body temperature.

Other women prefer more sophisticated methods to predict ovulation such as urine-based tests kits used to identify the surge in luteinizing hormone that occurs 12 to 48 hours before ovulation, or electronic fertility monitors, such as the OvaCue Fertility Monitor, a saliva-based test kit, that detects the steady increase of estrogen before ovulation.

The more sophisticated methods can be helpful but, bottom line, when trying to get pregnant, it is important to track cervical fluid to know when you are fertile and basal body temperature to confirm that ovulation has occurred.

Health Status Consultation

When questioning a female patient for infertility, therapists should pay close attention to their menstrual history as it offers the best clues to the person's condition. Aspects to focus on:

- Length of the menstrual cycle – either normal, short, long or irregular
- Premenstrual Syndrome (PMS)
- Dysfunctional Uterine Bleeding such as:
    - Heavy or prolonged bleeding or menorrhagia
    - Spotting during the menstrual cycle
    - Absences of periods or amenorrhea
    - Painful periods or dysmenorrhea
- Quality of the menstrual Blood such as the color, texture, odor plus clotting and length of the period
- Cervical secretion (See page 27)
- Changes in basil body temperature (See page 28)

Menstrual Cycle Patterns

The duration of the menstrual cycle can reveal a lot about the women's health and can indicate whether ovulation is occurring regularly. Irregular cycles often relate to a Liver and hormonal imbalance.

When a menstrual cycle lasts less than 21 days, ovulation is not occurring. This may be the result of a decrease in the number of eggs which stimulates the release of additional Follicle Stimulating Hormone (FSH). The increase in FSH leads to the early development of the follicle and earlier ovulation, thus shortening the menstrual cycle. Bleeding may occur even in the absence of ovulation.

Longer menstrual cycles that last more than 35 days are an indication that ovulation is either not occurring or that it occurs irregularly. High levels of stress can impede ovulation in women with normal-length menstrual cycles. Called silent anovulation, this condition can affect up to one-third of apparently normal menstrual cycles and can lead to an increased risk of bone density loss, early heart attack and breast cancer.

A women's menstrual cycle can be regular or menses may come:

Too Early from Blood Heat or Spleen Qi Deficiency
Too Late from a Cold Uterus, Kidney Yang Deficiency, Blood Deficiency or Qi Stagnation
Erratic from Liver Qi Stagnation or Kidney Deficiency

Too Early (Period comes before day 24)

Excess Heat
Blood is heavy, thick, dark red or purple red
Often accompanied by Liver Qi Stagnation with irritability and abdominal distension
Pulse: Rapid, Full
Tongue: Red with yellow coat
Tx: Clear Heat and cool Blood

Heat Stagnation
Flow can be heavy or light, but contains clots and dark Blood
Irritability
Shen disturbances
Pain in lower abdomen
Pulse: Wiry, rapid, full
Tongue: Dark, red
Tx: Dredge Liver to clear Heat. Strengthen the Spleen. Nourish the Blood

Spleen Qi Deficiency
Either heavy or light flow
Blood is light colored or clear
Sweating without exertion
Cold hands, feet or nose
Down-bearing sensation in the Uterus during menstrual cramps
Pulse: Thin, weak
Tongue: Pale with thin white coating. May be swollen
Tx: Tonify Qi and Strengthen the Spleen

Too Late (Longer than 28 to 33 days for three consecutive months. Can be 40 to 50 days between)

Excess Cold (Cold Uterus)
Blood is dark, not too heavy a flow
Lower abdomen pain with cold, relived by warmth
Pulse: Deep, Slow
Tongue: Normal
Tx: Warm the Uterus. Tonify Kidney Yang

Deficiency Cold (Kidney Yang Deficiency)
Blood is light in color, thin and clear in quality
Flow is not too heavy
Mild abdominal pain relieved by warmth
Pulse: Deep, Thin, May be slow
Tongue: Pale and/or swollen
Tx: Tonify Blood. Warm the Channels. Tonify Kidney Yang

Blood Deficiency
Light colored, thin, clear Blood with scanty flow
Dry skin
Fatigue
Dizziness
Pulse: Thin, Weak
Tongue: Pale
Tx: Boost Qi. Tonify Blood. Nourish Heart. Calm Shen

Qi Stagnation
Clots in menses
Abdominal distension
Abdominal pain
Irritability
Purple-colored Blood
Pulse: Choppy or Wiry
Tongue: Normal
Tx: Dredge the Liver. Move Blood. Regulate Menses

Erratic (Sometimes early, sometimes late, unpredictable. Usually due to dysregulation of Blood and Jing)

Liver Qi Stagnation
Menstrual Blood is thick and dark or purplish in color
Alternating heavy and light flow, with clots
Premenstrual symptoms including:
    Breast tenderness
    Irritability
    Lower abdomen pain
    Premenstrual bloating
    Headache
    Sleep disturbance
Pulse: Wiry, Thin
Tongue: Normal
Tx: Move Liver Qi and Blood. Calm the Mind

Kidney Qi Deficiency
Light flow, light in color, with lower back soreness
Possibly urinary frequency
Pulse: Thin, Weak
Tongue: Normal, or Pale or Thin
Tx: Tonify the Kidneys. Nourish Blood

Premenstrual Syndrome (PMS)

PMS is the most common gynecological problem experienced by women. PMS indicates Liver Qi Stagnation and Blood Stasis which is an Excess Pattern. Menstrual pain after the period indicates a Deficiency Pattern.

Some women only have mild symptoms, while some others suffer greatly. The symptoms vary from woman to woman, and each woman's symptoms may vary from month to month. Diagnosis is usually symptom based.

PMS symptoms may include anxiety, becoming easily angered, mood swings, breast swelling and tenderness, digestive disorders, headaches especially migraines, Heart palpitations, bitter taste and dry mouth.

Dysfunctional Uterine Bleeding

Dysfunctional Uterine Bleeding (DUB) is irregular, abnormal uterine bleeding that is not caused by a tumor, infection, or pregnancy. It is a disorder that occurs most frequently in women at the beginning and end of their reproductive lives.

About half the cases occur in women over 45 years of age, and about one fifth occur in women under the age of 20. Failure of the ovary to release an egg during the menstrual cycle occurs in about 70% of women with DUB.

Dysfunctional Uterine Bleeding is characterized by irregular periods, and excessive or prolonged menstrual flow. It can have many causes such as an unhealthy lifestyle, poor diet or improper eating habits, lack of exercise, environmental factors, emotional or psychological issues, toxins and hereditary influences.

Normally, abnormal bleeding is caused by a reduction in progesterone. If the follicle does not mature and ovulation does not occur, progesterone is not released. Therefore, in the continued presence of estrogen the lining of the Uterus continues to grow. The lining becomes thicker and unstable, outgrows its blood supply. It finally releases leading to bleeding that often will last for a longer period than normal.

DUB weakens the internal organs, affects Blood and Qi, and impairs the Conception and Penetrating Vessels, resulting in an uncontrollable menstrual flow.

When doing a consultation for Dysfunctional Uterine Bleeding, the acupuncturist will ask about the specific characteristics of the bleeding, including the duration, interval, amount of bleeding, color, odor and texture of the Blood, and the accompanying symptoms.

Women should see a doctor immediately if experiencing excruciating pain, nausea, vomiting and/or excessive bleeding at any point in the menstrual cycle. DUB resembles several other types of uterine bleeding disorders and sometimes overlaps these conditions.

Menorrhagia

For example, menorrhagia is menstrual periods with abnormally heavy or prolonged bleeding. Menstrual periods occur regularly, but last more than seven days, and blood loss exceeds 3 oz (88.7 ml). Passing blood clots is common.

This type of period can be a symptom of DUB, or many other diseases or disorders. Most women don't experience Blood loss severe enough to be defined as menorrhagia.

With heavy uterine bleeding, it is hard to build up the Blood. Heavy bleeding is tiring and depletes both progesterone and estrogen.

Some common causes of heavy bleeding or long periods include:
- Hormone imbalance
- Dysfunction of the ovaries
- Uterine fibroids or polyps
- Adenomyosis (Endometrium glands embed in the uterine muscle)
- Intrauterine Device (IUD)
- Pregnancy complications such as a miscarriage
- Cancer
- Inherited bleeding disorders
- Medications including anti-inflammatory medications, hormonal medications and anticoagulants.
- Other medical conditions such as Liver or Kidney disease.

Heavy bleeding or long periods in adolescent girls is typically due to anovulation. Adolescent girls are especially prone to anovulatory cycles in the first year after their first menstrual period.

In older reproductive-age women heavy bleeding or long periods is typically caused by uterine fibroids, polyps and adenomyosis. Other potential issues are uterine cancer, bleeding disorders, medication side effects and Liver or Kidney disease.

According to TCM, menorrhagia may be the result of:

- Spleen Qi Deficiency with inability to keep the Blood in the vessels
- Kidney Deficiency. Unable to astringe Jing, which forms Blood

- Blood Heat which forces the Blood out of the vessels
- Blood Stasis which inhibits the Blood vessels from constricting, allowing the Blood to escape

In addition to periods with abnormally heavy or prolonged bleeding, Uterine bleeding may include:

- Bleeding between periods
- Bleeding after sex
- Spotting anytime in the menstrual cycle
- Bleeding after menopause

Mid-cycle Spotting from Hormonal Imbalance

The hormones released throughout the menstrual cycle via the Hypothalamic-Pituitary-Ovarian Axis (HPO) regulate fertility. They regulate everything from growing the womb lining and follicles to ovulation and implantation of the embryo. Any type of disruption in this system may trigger mid-cycle spotting.

Mid-cycle Spotting During or After Ovulation

During the first half of the cycle, the hormone estrogen is predominant. This causes the lining of the Uterus to grow and thicken, in preparation for the implantation of the egg.

After ovulation progesterone levels gradually build up to hold the lining of the Uterus in place. When there is spotting or bleeding during ovulation the thickened lining of the Uterus has not been fully secured in place due to a deficiency of progesterone. A small amount of the womb lining may shed.

Bleeding from Failure to Ovulate

Mid-cycle bleeding may occur in a cycle where there is no ovulation due to a withdrawal of estrogen. Low estrogen levels mean that a surge of LH doesn't happen (LH triggers ovulation).

Therefore, ovulation does not occur, so progesterone cannot be secreted. A lighter or shorter period may be experienced sooner than the period is due.

Implantation Bleeding

This occurs when an embryo implants into the lining of the womb. This movement of the egg can result in light bleeding or spotting, which is completely normal and should not require medical attention.

In general, around a third of pregnant women will experience this. Implantation bleeding is typically light pink to dark brown (rust-colored), should not present any clots, and last anywhere from a couple of hours to three full days.

Mid-cycle spotting from Endometriosis

Women with endometriosis sometimes report mid-cycle spotting. The excess of endometrial tissue that builds up may slough off.

Rupture of an Ovarian Cyst

Rupture of an ovarian cyst may lead to abnormal uterine bleeding. Symptoms usually occur around the time that ovulation should happen such as sharp pain on either side of the lower abdomen and slight bleeding around the time of ovulation.

Abnormalities of the Cervix

Cervical abnormalities are rare. HPV (Human Papillomavirus, the most common sexually transmitted infection) or cervical fibroids may cause some slight bleeding mid-cycle. Very rarely, abnormalities of the cervix may be cancerous. Mid-cycle bleeding that is accompanied by pain in the cervical region, should be investigated by the patient's doctor.

Sexual Intercourse

Around the time of ovulation, the cervix becomes more sensitive. Sexual intercourse may cause some slight damage to the cervix, producing light bleeding. Mucous tinged with bright red Blood is common after sexual intercourse around the time of ovulation.

Bleeding After Menopause

In clinical terms, menopause occurs when a woman has not had a period for 12 months. Vaginal bleeding after menopause may be entirely harmless. However, it could result from something serious, so it's important the patient see her doctor promptly.

Uterine bleeding in menopausal women may be the result of Liver and Kidney Deficiency, or Spleen and Qi Deficiency often combined with Blood Stasis. Qi Deficiency weakens the blood vessels, so they are unable to contain the Blood. Excess Heat results in the reckless movement of hot Blood. Blood Stasis causes obstructions in the blood vessels forcing the Blood out of its normal pathways.

Amenorrhea

Amenorrhea is absence of periods or light, scanty periods. Examples are young women who haven't started menstruating by age 15 or women and girls who haven't had a period for 90 days, even if they haven't been menstruating for long.

Causes can include:
- Pregnancy
- Breastfeeding
- Extreme weight loss
- Eating disorders
- Excessive exercising
- Stress

Amenorrhea indicates a Blood Deficiency Pattern. The shorter, lighter periods may also point to the onset of menopause in older women or premature ovarian failure in younger women.

Amenorrhea can be a serious medical condition in need of treatment. In some cases, not having menstrual periods can mean the ovaries have stopped producing normal amounts of estrogen. Missing these hormones can have important effects on overall health. Hormonal problems may be caused by Polycystic Ovary Syndrome (PCOS) or serious problems with the reproductive organs.

In TCM, amenorrhea can be caused by unbalanced emotions, poor diet, Blood Deficiency, and invasions of pathogenic factors such as Dampness and Cold. The result is that Blood and Qi do not flow smoothly through the extra meridians, and do not reach the Uterus to form menses.

A patient with amenorrhea is much harder to treat but she can still get pregnant as the Blood gets more abundant.

Dysmenorrhea

Dysmenorrhea refers to cyclical abdominal pain including severe cramps which is experienced during or before menstruation. It occurs most typically in young women two to three years after the onset of menstruation.

Menstrual pain takes the form of cramping, lower abdominal pain, lower back pain or a pulling sensation in the inner thighs. Pain is often accompanied by headaches, dizziness, vomiting, nausea, diarrhea or constipation. Painful periods or menstrual cramps do not reflect on infertility.

Menstrual cramps in teens are caused by too much of a chemical called prostaglandin. Most teens with dysmenorrhea do not have a serious disease, even though the cramps can be severe.

In older women, the pain is sometimes caused by uterine fibroids, endometriosis or pelvic inflammatory disease. For some women, using a heating pad or taking a warm bath helps ease their cramps. Some over-the-counter pain medications can also help with these symptoms.

In Chinese medicine, painful menstrual cramps with sharp pain relieved after passing menstrual blood clots indicates a Blood Stasis Pattern. Dysmenorrhea with small, dark blood clots and abdominal pain indicates a Cold Pattern.

Menstrual pain, like other forms of pain, is caused by one or more of the following patterns:

- Qi Stagnation and Blood Stasis
- Qi and Blood Deficiency

- Excess Heat
- Dampness or Wind, or
- Imbalance of the Kidneys and Liver

Quality of Menstrual Blood

The quality of the menstrual Blood refers to its color, texture and odor. For example, thin, pale Blood points to a deficiency pattern while clotted, purplish Blood indicates the presence of an obstruction. Dark almost purplish Blood with large clots remains the major indicator of the presence of Blood Stasis in gynecological conditions.

The ideal color of menstrual Blood is bright red like the color of cranberries. The consistency is similar to Blood that bleeds from any other part of your body.

At the beginning or end of the period the Blood may be brown or dark red like the color of rust. Normally this is a sign that the discharged Blood is older.

Dark Red, Purplish Blood
Very dark almost purplish Blood with large clots points to Blood Stasis normally associated with Liver congestion. This can occur with conditions like endometriosis and fibroids and usually involves very intense, sharp, stabbing cramps and heavy flow.

Liver congestion is often accompanied by quite severe PMS symptoms such as headaches, breast distension and irritability. The Liver is easily affected by stress, so dark Blood tends to occur in women suffering from emotional stress.

Dark Blood with clots can also point to accumulation of Cold in the Uterus. There is not enough warmth to move the Blood. Dark Blood means that there is old stagnant Blood in the Uterus which stops fresh new Blood from being generated which is key to the health of the next menstrual cycle.

Deep-Red Color
A deep-red color that is thick in consistency accompanied by early, heavy periods (earlier than 24 days) indicates too much heat in the body and the possible presence of infection. If accompanied by other symptoms such as a fever, foul smelling discharge, or severe pelvic pain, the patient should consult her doctor immediately to check for infection.

Pale Blood
Pale pink Blood, especially with a watery consistency indicates deficiency of Spleen Qi. The flow can be very heavy or very light. Pale Blood which is also scanty can indicate a thin uterine lining.

Length of Menses

A short or delayed period is a sign of Blood Deficiency. A short or early period indicates Blood Heat. A longer than normal period points to Spleen Qi Deficiency. Irregular menstrual flow is indicative of Liver Qi Stagnation.

An early period can indicate the presence of Heat, a late period the accumulation of Cold in the Uterus, and irregular periods Qi Deficiency or Dampness in the Uterus. A strong odor emanating from the Blood is a symptom of Damp Heat.

Specific Questions to Ask

- How long have you been trying to get pregnant?
- Have you been pregnant in the past?
- Have you suffered any miscarriages?
- Have you used contraception before or an Intrauterine Device?
- Do you suffer from PMS? (Abdominal Pain, Breast Tenderness, Mood Swings)
- How long is the menstrual cycle?
- How long does menstrual bleeding last?
- Describe the menstrual Blood: Color, Texture, Smell
- Are the periods light, normal or heavy?
- Are there any Blood clots?

- Are the periods painful and if yes how many days does the pain last?
- Do you bleed or spot between periods?
- Have you undergone an IUI or InVitro cycle?
- Have you had Fibroids, Cysts, Endometriosis, STDs or any vaginal infections?
- Have you been diagnosed with pelvic adhesions or other abnormalities?
- How are your lifestyle habits (exercise, stress, caffeine, alcohol, smoking cigarettes)?
- How is your daily nutrition (vegetables, legumes, fruits, seeds, dairy products, sugars, fats, meat, seafood)?
- What medications do you take (prescribed, un-prescribed, over-the-counter)?
- Have you been exposed to any environmental toxins or hormones?
- Has your male partner had his sperm tested?
- What medication does your male partner take?
- Has your male partner had any infections, surgeries, or hernias?
- If necessary is he willing to undergo treatment with acupuncture and herbal medicine?

When differentiating the patterns of infertility look at the tongue, take the pulse, and note the associated signs and symptoms. A deep, slippery pulse is a clear sign of pregnancy. During ovulation the Kidney Yin pulse tends to rise from its usually deep level to the surface, bubbling up like a fountain.

Establishing Expectations

TCM's effectiveness has been recognized by The World Health Organization in the treatment of over 40 common disorders including allergies, anxiety, depression, infertility, insomnia, and migraines.

In 2016, the Complementary Therapies in Medicine Journal published a review showing that women were twice as likely to conceive within four months of using Chinese herbal medicine treatments compared to those who opted for IVF or conventional Western medical fertility drug treatment. The results showed as well that the quality of a woman's menstrual cycle seems to be a vital factor for the successful treatment of female infertility.

There are several theories as to why Chinese medicine can be beneficial to fertility rates, including the possibility that herbal remedies and acupuncture can:

- Regulate the ovulation and menstrual cycle
- Enhance Blood flow to the Uterus
- Enhance endorphin production calming the central nervous system
- Regulate and balance the hormones by affecting the Hypothalamic-Pituitary-Ovarian Axis

Why is acupuncture so effective?

Blood flow, Blood flow, Blood flow! This is how every single cell in our bodies are nourished. Treatments help patients enjoy a deep state of relaxation, taking them out of the fight or flight mode, and encouraging blood flow to the internal organs.

Some practitioners claim a 30% success rate in treating infertility with acupuncture for patients younger than 39 years of age, and an 85% success rate when acupuncture is combined with herbal medicine after eight months of treatment. Regardless of acupuncture's proven effectiveness, guarantees of success should never be provided as each patient reacts differently to treatment.

Treatment Frequency

Patients want to know what kind of commitment is required to treatment in both time and money. Most of the women treated fall into the once a week category for a minimum of three months and for up to a year.

Determining treatment frequency depends on many factors. Do patients need to come twice a week?

Probably not unless there is something more significant going on, like overgrowth of reproductive tissue. Endometriosis for example would require more frequent treatment. It is the leading cause of infertility in women.

Treatment frequency truly does depend on:
- Where the patient is in the process
- What specific difficulties they are experiencing
- How they respond to treatment

To help regulate the menstrual cycle acupuncture and herbal medicine treatments are provided in each of the four phases: Menstrual, Follicular, Ovulation and Luteal Phases. These treatments balance the hormonal system and reinforce the body's natural reproductive cycle.

Treatment must also address specific issues emotional or physical identified by the process of pattern differentiation.

Most Important Times for Acupuncture

Although treatments normally follow the phases of the women's menstrual cycle the most important times for acupuncture are:

- During the follicular phase - Day 5, 6, 7 or 8 of the menstrual cycle
- The day of, day before or day after ovulation (as indicated by the LH surge)
- During implantation time (6 - 10 days after ovulation)

Treatment plans for men require weekly acupuncture and Chinese herbs for a minimum of three months. The treatment focuses primarily on improving the quality of the sperm.

Every time a patient undergoes a treatment, its effects accumulate bringing about a little more balance inside the body. With better balance, the chances of conceiving are optimized.

Often the requirements of treatment must be coordinated with the availability of the patient. When determining treatment frequency remember that acupuncture is a process-oriented method of medical intervention. It is better to do more than less.

Regulating the Menstrual Cycle

Classic Chinese gynecological medicine emphasizes the regulation of the menstrual cycle as a means of improving internal balance and treating common and often complex women's health complaints.

This approach was developed largely by Professor Xia Gui Cheng of the Nanjing University of Traditional Chinese Medicine in China. According to Professor Cheng the menstrual cycle has four phases.

Day 1 to 5 - Menstrual Phase
Day 5 to 11 - Pre-Ovulation or Follicular Phase
Day 11 to 15 - Ovulation Phase or Mid-Cycle
Day 15 to 28 - Post-Ovulation or Luteal Phase

Each of these phases requires different treatment methods according to what is happening in the body during the respective phase. It is important to do a detailed diagnosis of the patient's individual pattern of disharmony. The patient is then treated according to her individual pattern of disharmony and the phase of the menstrual cycle.

Although 28 days is considered the norm for the length of a menstrual cycle, menstrual phases can stretch and contract from 25 to 34 days. Cycles of women suffering from Polycystic Ovarian Syndrome can last from two to three months. For the first few years after the onset of menstruation, longer cycles are common. A woman's cycle tends to shorten and become more regular with age.

The beginning of each phase of an irregular cycle can still be identified:

- Phase 1 starts with the first full day of menstrual bleeding.
- Phase 2 starts with the end of bleeding.
- Phase 3 is identified by a change in cervical secretion and an increase in basal body temperature.
- Phase 4 can often be detected by the appearance of premenstrual symptoms.

Menstrual Phase - Day 1 to 5

Generally, day 1 of the cycle is the first day of significant menstrual bleeding, not just spotting. If the period begins in the evening or during the night, from about 6 p.m. to midnight, day 1 is the following day.

This phase is characterised by the downward movement of Qi and Blood. The activity is centered on the central abdomen below the umbilicus and is under the influence of the Chong Mai and the descending of Heart Qi for the discharge of menstrual Blood. Insufficient discharge at this point in the cycle may lead to retention of the menses and possibly the development of endometriosis.

On average menses will last from 4 to 6 days, and possibly up to 7 days. The Blood should be a fresh red color, with no clotting or smell. The Blood is neither diluted nor thick. The color is light red in the beginning, dark red in the middle of the menses and lighter red or pinkish towards the end. The flow of Blood starts with a trickle, flows more abundantly in the middle, to end with a trickle.

Menstrual health depends on the amount of Qi in the Ren and Chong Vessels where all the Qi and Blood meet. In women, both channels begin in the space between the Kidneys and have domain over the Uterus. The Du Mai or Governing Channel also starts in the space between the Kidneys. A healthy menstrual cycle requires Du and Ren to be in balance.

A quick drop in progesterone usually precedes the beginning of the period, and on day 1 both the estrogen and progesterone levels are relatively low. Yang is at its maximum at the onset and decreases rapidly, transforming into Yin. The sharp drop in Yang usually signals the disappearance of PMS. The invasion of the Uterus by Cold, Damp or Heat occurs most often during menstruation, pregnancy or the postnatal period.

During menstruation, the endometrial lining of the Uterus is shed. The lining should be fully expelled and Qi and Blood stagnation in the Uterus cleared. The clearing of the endometrial lining is very important for the development of a new, thick endometrial layer, a necessary component of successful conception.

From a Chinese medicine point of view, with the loss of Blood during menstruation the Ren and Chong gradually empty, and by the time the menses is over the Ren and Chong, Kidney Yin and Liver Blood, are at their lowest levels in the cycle.

Problems during the menstrual period are mostly related to Stagnation of Qi and Blood, while problems that occur or are worse towards the end of the menses are generally associated with Blood Deficiency.

Some practitioners will use herbs to "flush" the uterine lining during menstruation, encouraging the complete discharge of the endometrium, even if there are no overt symptoms of Blood Stasis. If there are signs of stasis, such as clotting, cramping, or irregular bleeding, this may be a particularly useful strategy.

A typical base formula used during this stage is Jia Wei Tao Hong Si Wu Tang or Chong Release Formula. This formula is especially effective in treating menstrual Blood Stasis. It opens the collaterals to eliminate Blood Stasis and facilitates the complete discharge of the endometrial lining.

The main goal of acupuncture treatment is to nourish and invigorate Blood, or reduce bleeding if the period is heavy, eliminate Stasis, scatter Cold, and warm the Uterus. Once bleeding subsides after a few days into the menses, the treatment can shift to nourishing Yin and Blood.

Pre-ovulation or Follicular Phase - Days 5 to 11

The follicular phase starts on day 1 of the menstrual cycle when new follicles, containing eggs, begin their growth. Clinically, the support of this phase generally begins after the major menstrual Blood flow is over, usually around day 4.

From a Chinese medical perspective, follicle development is a Yin process, dependent on Yin, Blood and Essence. Therefore, it is important during this period to treat any Deficiency of Yin or Blood. Yin and Blood deficiency affecting fertility may manifest with poor follicular development, thin endometrial lining, or decreased cervical mucus.

The regeneration of the endometrium, or uterine lining, begins about two days after the onset of menstruation, even though menstrual bleeding continues. This process includes tissue repair of the Uterus where the lining has shed as well as the development of estrogen and progesterone receptors in the new tissue.

This phase is important in establishing a good menstrual cycle. It represents the crossroads of Yin and Yang when Yin is beginning to grow. Yin and Blood gradually build to fill the Ren and Chong Meridians. The ovarian follicles are growing, estrogen levels are rising. basal body temperatures remain relatively low.

The hypothalamus and the pituitary glands interact, stimulating the pituitary to release FSH (Follicle Stimulating Hormone) to recruit follicles in preparation for ovulation. One of these follicles will grow to become the largest, or dominant follicle, and will release its egg at ovulation.

Estrogen is the dominant hormone during this phase. As the estrogen levels gradually rise it stimulates the proliferation and thickening of the endometrium and its dense vascular network, and an increase in fertile mucus necessary to escort the sperm through the cervix for fertilization of the released eggs.

Heat may be a problem during this phase, as it easily damages Yin, and can enter the Blood prompting it to move recklessly at ovulation or menstruation. Heat can also cause follicles to grow too quickly resulting in poor egg quality and may cause early ovulation and the shortening of the entire menstrual cycle. Heat in the follicular phase is commonly due to Yin Deficiency or stagnation of Heart and Liver Qi.

Patients with fertility problems frequently experience a great deal of stress when month after month they are unable to conceive. In these cases, Heat from emotional stagnation may disturb the steady building of Yin and Blood, and is often seen in upward spikes in the basal body temperature.

Gui Shao Di Huang Wan sometimes called Nourish Ren and Chong Formula is a very effective formula for this stage to help regulate the length of the Follicular Phase, increase cervical mucus, improve the quality and quantity of menstrual Blood, regulate basal body temperature, and improve the development of follicles and the endometrial lining.

The Heart and Liver may be addressed with additions or modifications to the formula. This phase is very important in cases of infertility when there is a delayed ovulation, thin endometrium, decreased cervical mucus, and poor quality or number of eggs.

With the use of Yin and Blood tonic herbs, fertility signs often show clear improvement. Long or short follicular phases regulate, cervical mucus increases, menstrual Blood quantity and quality improves, and basal body temperature charts become more even. Western tests often show improvement in follicle and endometrial lining development.

The main goal of acupuncture treatment is to nourish and move Blood, by warming and tonifying Kidney Yang and tonifying Spleen Qi, tonify Kidney Yin, and sooth Liver Qi.

Ovulation or Mid-Cycle Phase - Day 11 to 15

A woman's most fertile time is during ovulation, which typically occurs within day 11 through day 21, counting from the first day of a woman's period. The 11th day is most likely the earliest day a woman will ovulate. The 21st day is most likely the last.

Chong, Ren and Du are in full activity to promote ovulation. Yin is at its maximum. Yang begins to rise. It is a dynamic time, one in which the menstrual energy transitions from the Yin half of the cycle to the Yang half. A strong movement of Qi and Blood allows for the transition to occur with subsequent expulsion of the egg from the follicle.

Activity is centered around the lateral sides of the lower abdomen, which are under the influence of the Chong Mai. The beginning of this phase is indicated by the appearance of a viscous, transparent, clear, stretchy secretion produced by the cervix indicating imminent ovulation.

Normally the greatest amount of cervical secretion is produced the day of ovulation with maximum Yin. Immediately following ovulation, the cervical secretion thickens. Kidney Deficiency may be present if the cervical secretion is absent or short-lasting.

Prior to ovulation, the hypothalamus and pituitary gland play a major role as LH (Luteinizing Hormone) is released. This causes the LH Surge which occurs about 24 hours prior to ovulation as detected by an ovulation predictor kit.

When the main developing follicle becomes large enough and estrogen reaches a certain level, ovulation will occur. As Yin changes to Yang, activity and movement are expressed as the dominant egg bursts from the follicle.

The process of ovulation is dependent on the strength and fullness of Yin, the ability to mobilize Yang, and the movement of Qi and Blood to facilitate transition. Growth of Yin must be exuberant to induce the Yang movement of ovulation. Ovulation occurs with a quick change of Yin to Yang.

In a normal, healthy ovulation, the basal body temperature chart will show a slight drop followed by a quick rise in temperature with the LH surge, and temperatures will then stay relatively high throughout the second half of the cycle.

During the ovulation phase, if Yin does not decrease or if Yang does not increase, Dampness and Phlegm may invade the Uterus causing obstruction, possibly delaying ovulation. Yin Deficiency or Yang Excess may lead to early ovulation. Long or irregular cycles, the absence of periods, pain at ovulation, basal body temperatures that are not biphasic may indicate problems with the transitional movement.

The Heart is also involved in ovulation through the activity of the Bao Mai, the collateral connecting the Heart to the Uterus. The Bao Mai is one of the pathways by which the action of the Heart Qi and Blood descend to the reproductive organs, keeping them nourished and facilitating movement.

The main goal of treatment is to promote ovulation and encourage healthy Qi by nourishing Essence, tonifying Kidney Yang, warming the Uterus and strengthening Ren and Chong. If needed resolve Dampness and tonify the Spleen.

Bu Shen Cu Pai Luan sometimes called Jade Moon Phase 3 is a commonly used formula for mid-cycle support. The formula invigorates the Blood and removes stasis, while promoting a healthy Yin foundation and the ability for Yang to mobilize at ovulation.

Herbs during this phase of the cycle are generally administered about three days before ovulation, or when ovulation should ideally occur, until two days after ovulation.

Post-Ovulation or Luteal Phase - Days 15 to 28

After the egg is released at ovulation, the sperm and egg travel to meet in the fallopian tubes, where a successful sperm will penetrate and fertilize the egg. The egg must be fertilized in the fallopian tubes within about 12 hours of ovulation. Then it continues moving to the Uterus to implant in the endometrial lining. Implantation begins about seven days after ovulation. Progesterone levels rise. BBT temperatures are ideally at least 4/10 of a degree higher than in the Follicular Phase.

Qi and Yang are dominant with Yang rising rapidly and approaching its maximum. Fertilization and conception are dependent on the dynamic action of Yang which supports movement and activity. Yang gives warmth to the Uterus to eliminate Yin pathogenic factors such as Blood Stasis, Cold and Phlegm. The Chong Vessel also exerts a strong influence on this phase.

After ovulation, the Corpus Luteum is formed at the site on the ovary wall where the follicle released its egg. The Corpus Luteum is the remains of the ovarian follicle that has released a mature ovum during ovulation. It is a temporary endocrine structure involved in the production of high levels of progesterone to:

- Keep the endometrium rich in hormones and nutrients
- Maintain a healthy environment for implantation.
- Inhibit the development of new eggs

Progesterone is the key hormone in the luteal phase of the cycle and is evident in the higher basal body temperatures. The luteal phase is dominated by Qi and Yang but is also dependent on a good foundation of Yin and Blood.

For implantation to occur, the uterine lining or endometrium must be healthy and receptive. The endometrium must be thick, moist, and rich in Blood and nutrients, a very Yin environment in which the fertilized egg burrows until it is completely buried by the end of the cycle Problems with the luteal phase may been seen in:

- Significant drops in basal body temperatures in the second half of the cycle
- Progesterone insufficiency
- Problems with implantation
- Tendency to miscarriage

Pre-menstrual symptoms may appear caused by Liver Qi Stagnation, Yang excess from Liver Fire or Heart Fire, or Yang Deficiency from Spleen Yang or Kidney Yang Deficiency. Although pre-menstrual tension is not itself an indicator of infertility, it may compound the difficulty, so addressing the organ systems involved may be employed as a secondary treatment principle to help move Qi and Blood.

In fertility treatments, ideally the Yin and Blood were already well nourished in the follicular phase and cleared of stasis in the menstrual phase.

In the luteal phase, it is appropriate to continue supporting Yin and Blood, while tonifying Yang, move Qi and Blood to help expel Cold and resolve Dampness, normalize Liver Qi, and warm the Uterus.

In Chinese gynecology, it is common practice to support Yin when treating the Yang. Tonifying Yin supports the foundation or root of the Yang and protects the Yin from the warming nature of Yang.

Do not open the Ren and Penetrating vessels after ovulation as this could cause a miscarriage. The energy is already built up and will naturally release with a normal period.

Jian Gu Tang sometimes called Yuan Support Formula supports the luteal phase well by tonifying and invigorating the Yang and the Spleen Qi. The formula is often modified with herbs to support the Yin and Blood, to move Liver Qi stagnation, and calm the Spirit.

Protocols to Regulate the Menstrual Cycle

According to Jake Paul Fratkin, OMD, of AcupunctureToday.com, Chinese medicine delineates several patterns of infertility. In most cases, supplementation of Blood and Kidney Qi is necessary. Further pattern differentiation can be made such as Deficiency of Kidney Yang, Yin or Jing; Liver Qi Stagnation, Blood Stasis, Cold in the Uterus, or accumulation of Phlegm and Dampness.

Remember that in identifying patterns of disharmony, paying close attention to the menstrual history offers the best clues. Irregular periods or premenstrual syndrome (irritability, breast distension, abdominal distension) indicate Qi stagnation; dysmenorrhea or painful menstrual cramps indicates Blood Stasis or a Cold Uterus; amenorrhea or light, scanty periods point to Blood Deficiency; and obesity involves stagnation of Phlegm and Dampness.

Ultimately the goal of treatment is to clear obstructions in the Uterus and increase the flow of Blood to the reproductive organs.

Many different acupuncture points are used to enhance fertility in both men and women. Based on traditional diagnostic techniques, different acupuncturists may choose different acupuncture points depending on each patient's presenting symptoms and constitutional patterns.

One if not the most important aspect of fertility treatments is the regulation of the menstrual cycle.

Pathologies such as Endometriosis, Uterine Fibroids, Ovarian Cysts, Accumulation of Cold or Damp in the Uterus, and Pelvic Inflammatory Disease may be treated for two to three menstrual cycles or until notable progress is achieved before focusing on the normalization of the menstrual cycle.

When regulating the menstrual cycle, the primary pattern should always be addressed no matter what phase is being treated.

The different phases of the menstrual cycle such as follicle maturation, ovulation, shedding and growth of the endometrium, and the maturation of the ova and corpus luteum reflect the movement of Kidney Yin and Kidney Yang.

Phase 1: Menstrual Phase (Day 1 to 5)

Menstruation is the reproductive system's time to rest. According to Randine Lewis, Ph.D. in Oriental Medicine and author of The Infertility Cure, the state of the menses reflects the health of the hormonal activity of the ovaries. With a healthy period:

- The menstrual flow is smooth and neither scanty or excessive
- The color of the Blood is red, not brown or black
- The consistency of Blood should not be watery
- Clots are minimal to none
- Bleeding lasts approximately 4 to 6 days then stops without spotting
- There is no uterine, abdominal or lower back pain

Problems Encountered During the Menstrual Phase

When the reproductive system is not functioning properly, possible issues encountered during the menstrual phase may include Blood Stasis or Blood Deficiency, Qi Stagnation or Deficiency, or excess Heat from Liver Qi Stagnation or Yin Deficiency.

Symptoms	Indications
A sharp or stabbing pain	Blood Stasis
A dull or heavy aching pain	Qi Deficiency
Bloating or distention	Qi Stagnation
Scanty Blood flow or short period (1 to 2 days)	Insufficient Blood to nourish the uterine lining. Often corresponds to a lack of estrogen in the Follicular Phase.
Pink & watery Blood	Spleen Qi Deficiency
Scant & brownish Blood	Blood Deficiency & Blood Stasis
Heavy Blood flow lasting beyond seven days or occurs outside of menses	Insufficient Qi to control the menstrual cycle. Possible Spleen Qi Deficiency.
Heavy painful flow with dark & clotty Blood	Blood Stasis: Obstructed Blood stagnates & oxidizes becoming dark, clotty & painful creating a toxic environment in the Uterus

Profuse, bright red Blood with a short menstrual cycle & other Heat signs.	Excess Heat. May involve Liver Qi Stagnation or Yin Deficiency.
Absence of menses (Amenorrhea)	Blood Deficiency or not enough Blood or Blood Stasis blocking menstruation

In the Menstrual Phase Qi and Blood are descending. The main goal of treatment is to ensure the complete discharge of the endometrial lining which paves the way for the growth of a new uterine lining allowing for proper implantation and placental development. This is achieved by invigorating the Blood to eliminate Blood Stasis.

Stagnation in the Uterus caused by accumulation of Cold or Damp may need to be addressed. If the period is heavy, it may be necessary to reduce Blood flow by tonifying Qi, clearing Heat or resolving Blood Stasis.

Once bleeding subsides at about Day 4 of a 28-day cycle, the focus of treatment shifts to nourishing Kidney Yin and Blood.

Points	Effect
SP 4 Right & PC 6 Left (Always open the extraordinary vessels for 10 minutes before adding additional needles).	Moves Blood by opening & regulating the Chong Mai which has domain over menstruation. Treats PMS, painful, heavy & irregular periods, accumulation of Phlegm & Endometriosis. Calms the Spirit in hormonal disorders. SP 4 has a calming effect on the womb & can be safely stimulated during pregnancy. PC 6 calms the Mind.
LU 7 Right & Kid 6 Left With Ren 4 nourishes the Kidneys. With Ren 6 moves Qi in the lower abdomen.	Opens the Ren channel helping to regulate the period & hormonal imbalances affecting the Uterus. Treats irregular, absent & late periods. Tonifies the Uterus & Ovaries. Influences the fluid metabolism.

SP 6 With Ren 4 opens the Uterus & encourages the strong & smooth downward movement of the menstrual flow.	By regulating the Spleen, Liver & Kidney channels, SP 6 treats all gynecological disorders of the lower abdomen related to Blood Stasis, Kidney Deficiency, Phlegm-Dampness or Liver Qi Stagnation. Treats irregular menstruation & uterine bleeding, amenorrhea, menorrhagia, dysmenorrhea, & difficult labor. Tonifies Spleen Qi & Yang, strengthening its ability to hold the Blood.
SP 8 (Xi-Cleft Point)	Resolves Blood Stasis in the Uterus & lower abdomen. Treats irregular menstruation, dysmenorrhea & abdominal masses in women from Qi & Blood Stasis.
SP 10	Moves, supplements & cools Blood. Treats irregular menstruation, amenorrhea, dysmenorrhea, uterine bleeding with or without Blood clots. Controls the extent of bleeding if there is Heat.
BL 17 (Diaphragm Shu)	Resolves bleeding disorders related mainly to Blood Stasis & Heat primarily for the Lungs & Stomach. Nourishes Blood & Yin. Treats Blood Deficiency caused by Blood Stasis.
St 28	This point has a very ancient history of use for infertility to treat Blood Stasis, Damp & Phlegm conditions. Always combine with **Kid 14,** a point of the Chong Mai & a major point to move Blood.
Kid 14 Most important point on the Chong Mai for moving Blood.	Regulates Qi & Blood. Resolves Blood Stasis in the Uterus. Treats irregular menses, dysmenorrhea, uterine bleeding, & abdominal pain.

Kid 5	Regulates Qi & Blood in the Kidney, Ren & Chong channels. Treats irregular menstruation, amenorrhea, dysmenorrhea, delayed menstruation from Qi or Blood Deficiency or Blood Stasis.
Kid 8	Resolves Blood Stasis. Stops uterine bleeding primarily from Kidney Deficiency & Blood Stasis, Blood Heat & Damp Heat. Treats irregular menstruation, amenorrhea & dysmenorrhea.
SP 8 & LI 4	Treat acute dysmenorrhea or painful menstruation with cramps
Liv 8	Reduces Blood Stasis in the Uterus, abdominal masses & pain, & amenorrhea. Clears Damp Heat from the Lower Jiao. Damp Heat & Blood Stasis are common gynecological disorders.
LI 4 (Often used with Liv 3 to move Qi & open the body.)	Encourages the upward & downward movement of Qi. Relieves pain conditions.
Liv 3, GB 34, GB 41	Moves Liver Qi & removes stagnation
Ren 4 (Uterine Point)	Tonifies & moves Blood. Warms the Uterus. Supplements the Kidneys Yin & Yang. Nourishes Jing. Opens Chong & Ren.
Ren 5 (San Jiao Mu Point)	Stops bleeding. Tonifies Original Qi.
Ren 6	Supplements, regulates & holds the Qi helping moderate the downward movement of the menstrual flow. With **Kid 2** treats Cold/Qi Deficiency type of infertility.
Ren 7 (Yin Meeting point of Kidneys, Ren & Chong)	Treats infertility from any etiology due to the close relationship of the Kidneys, Ren & Chong with the Uterus. Treats uterine bleeding,

	irregular menstruation, amenorrhea & leucorrhoea.
SP 6, St 36, BL 20 (Spleen Shu), BL 21 (Stomach Shu)	Tonify Spleen Qi & nourishes Blood
SP 6 & Kid 3	Supplement Kidney Yin
Liv 2, Kid 2	Cool Blood & clear Heat
SP 1, SP 6, Ren 7, SJ 4	Treat uterine Bleeding
Kid 8, BL 55	Treat uterine Bleeding from Qi Deficiency
SP 6, Kid 8, Kid 10, Liv 3	Treat excessive uterine Bleeding (Heavy or prolonged menstrual bleeding)
Liv 1	Treats excessive uterine bleeding, menorrhagia & metrorrhagia (irregular bleeding especially between periods). Regulates Qi in the Lower Jiao.
SP 6, HT 5, Liv 2	Treat menorrhagia or abnormally heavy or prolonged menstrual bleeding.
ST 25 (LI Mu Point), ST 44	Clear Stomach Heat & calm digestion, acute diarrhea & constipation.
Tituo (Located 4 cun lateral to the midline level with Ren 4)	Regulates the Qi in the Uterus & moderates the descending action of SP 6. Treats dysmenorrhea, abdominal distention & pain. Combined with Du 20, St 36 & SP 6 treats prolapse of the Uterus.
PC 5	Makes Blood flow smoothly. Regulates the Uterus, relaxes ligaments & tendons, calms the Mind & helps stop vomiting.
BL 32	Regulates Qi in the Uterus. Invigorates Blood. Treats irregular menses & dysmenorrhea.

Phase 2: Follicular Phase (Day 5 to 11)

The main goal of this phase is to ensure healthy follicular development. During the Follicular Phase the egg matures to its fullest potential for release and fertilization, and the lining of the Uterus prepares for successful embryo implantation. The proper functioning of the Follicular Phase also influences the quality of the upcoming menses.

If the endometrium has not been fully discharged evidence of Blood Stasis may appear such as continued spotting of dark Blood after the period or a continued high BBT after the arrival of menses. If this is the case acupuncture points may be added to treat Blood Stasis.

At the beginning of the phase the focus is on building Kidney Yin. Combine acupuncture with herbs and meditation exercises to nourish Yin. Normally Kidney Yang is strengthened in the second half of the menstrual cycle when the Yin base is well established.

A longer Menstrual and Follicular Phase which together may last more than 15 days with a low BBT indicates a delayed or weak ovulation. This may reflect low estrogen levels or Kidney Yin Deficiency coupled with weak communication between the HPO axis and the ovaries which struggle to respond to signals from the brain to develop ovarian follicles and eggs.

Liver Qi Stagnation tends to cause more problems later in the cycle. But if the patient suffers from stress or pain during ovulation acupuncture points can be added to help pacify Heart and Liver Fire.

When dealing with Damp-Phlegm, supplementation of Yin and Yang should be approximately equal to avoid the risks of reinforcing Yin in a damp environment. By Day 9 of a 28-day cycle or when there are some signs of vaginal discharge or moisture, the focus of treatment shifts to moving Qi and Blood in preparation for ovulation. Supplementing Yang also helps prevent accumulation of Damp.

Anti-sperm antibodies in the cervical mucus reflect a subtle level of Blood Stasis. Regulating the Blood will help reduce the levels of antibodies allowing the sperm to enter the Uterus.

Clomiphene, a synthetic nonsteroidal drug, can be very effective in stimulating ovulation. But women who suffer from Yin Deficiency, as expressed by the lack of fertile mucus and thinning of the endometrium, may experience a decline in their condition with the use of this drug due to its anti-estrogen action.

Problems Encountered During the Follicular Phase

Symptoms	Indications
Low BBT in Follicular Phase	Generalized Yang Deficiency
Longer Phase	Spleen Qi Deficiency with or without Dampness or Deficiency of Kidney Jing, Yin or Blood
Shorter Phase - High BBT	Excess Heat normally from Kidney Yin Deficiency
Longer Phase - High BBT	Kidney Yin Deficiency
Longer Phase - Low BBT	Kidney Yang Deficiency
High BBT in Follicular Phase Initially	Obstruction of transformation from Yang to Yin
Unstable Follicular Phase BBT	Liver or Heart Fire

Normally Kidney Jing Deficiency must be addressed after the menses leading up to ovulation and during ovulation.

After menstruation the Chong and Ren Mai are depleted and must be built back up. Therefore, treatment focuses on regulating the Chong and Ren, nourishing and moving Blood, warming and tonifying Kidney Yin and Spleen Qi, and soothing Liver Qi. As Yin levels grow, Yang is consumed, so after Day 8 or 9 if ovulation is expected on Day 14, supplement Kidney Yang.

Points	Effect
SP 4 Right & PC 6 Left SP 4 has a calming effect on the womb & can be safely stimulated during pregnancy. PC 6 calms the Heart Fire with HT 5.	Moves Blood by opening & regulating the Chong Mai which has complete domain over menstruation. Calms the Spirit in hormonal disorders.

Lu 7 Right & Kid 6 Left With Ren 4 nourishes the Kidneys. With Ren 6 moves Qi in the lower abdomen.	Opens the Ren channel helping to regulate the period & hormonal imbalances affecting the Uterus. Tonifies the Uterus & Ovaries. Influences the fluid metabolism.
Ren 7, Kid 5, Kid 8, Kid 13	Balance Ren & Chong at the beginning of the Follicular Phase. Ren 7 & Kid 5 regulate the Uterus. Kid 5 invigorates Blood.
SP 4, ST 30	Influence the Chong Mai. ST 30 builds & invigorates Blood & disperses Cold & stagnation in the Uterus. SP 4 is a Chong Mai Master Point
ST 27	Influences Kidney Jing. Gathers & supplements Yin.
Ren 4	Tonifies & warms the Uterus. Supplements Kidney Yin, Yang & Jing. Builds Blood.
Ren 6	Fosters original Qi. Tonifies Yang. Helps move Qi & Blood.
Ren 7	Regulates the Uterus. Tonifies the Kidneys & Kidney Yin.
Kid 7, Du 4, Ren 6, BL 23, BL 32	Supplement Kidney Yang
Kid 3, Kid 6, SP 6, Ren 4	Supplement Kidney Yin
Ren 6, Ren 12, SP 6, SP 10, St 36, BL 20 (Spleen Shu), BL 21 (Stomach Shu)	Build Blood & supplement Spleen Qi. Ren 6 & St 36 strongly tonify Qi.
Ren 3, SP 6, SP 8, SP 10, SP 12, Liv 5, Liv 8, Kid 14, ST 29 & BL 17 (Diaphragm Shu)	Move, nourish, cool & harmonize Blood in gynecological disorders.
Ren 6, ST 36, GB 26	Move Qi & Blood

LI 4	Circulates Qi in the Uterus to help prevent cramping. Only use before ovulation as can stimulate uterine contractions.
With Liv 3 strongly moves Qi in whole body.	
Zi Gong	Brings Qi & Blood to the Uterus. Regulates menstruation.
Liv 2, HT 5, HT 7, PC 6, PC 7	Pacify Heart & Liver Fire

Phase 3: Ovulation or Mid-Cycle Phase (Day 11 to 15)

Yin and Blood have been replenished. The cervix is full of stretchy mucus. The ovary is ready to release a mature egg around day 13 or 14 of a 28-day cycle. At this very dynamic moment of the cycle Liver Qi transforms Yin (estrogen) into Yang (progesterone).

The beginning of this phase can be identified by the appearance of cervical secretion and a slight drop in temperature just prior to ovulation followed by a rise of about half of one-degree Fahrenheit or about one quarter of one-degree Celsius.

The basic treatment approach is to invigorate Qi and Blood. For patients suffering from a Phlegm-Damp condition Qi and Blood need to be moved well before ovulation for example on day 9 of a 28-day cycle or with the first signs of vaginal discharge or moisture, or the egg may never be released. Even if it is released its movement may be obstructed by excess mucus in the fallopian tubes.

Liver and Heart Qi must remain unobstructed for ovulation to occur. Bloating, sore breasts or nipples, and irritability at ovulation are signs of Liver Qi Stagnation. Delayed, scanty or absence of periods, mid-cycle spotting, and extreme restlessness or manic behavior indicates possible Heat in the Heart. Pain at ovulation is a sign of Blood Stasis.

The main goal of treatment is to reduce obstructions to ovulation and promote endometrial development by moving Qi and Blood. In addition, the treatment may also focus on tonifying Kidney Yang, warming the Uterus, strengthening Ren and Chong and calming the Mind. Phlegm-Damp conditions may need to be addressed.

If Yang does not rise sharply in the ovulatory phase and Qi and Blood do not move well, the egg may not be released, the tube may not successfully capture it or the Luteal Phase may be inadequate.

Points	Effect
Ren 6, GB 26, SP 5, BL 28	Move Qi & Blood
SP 4	Regulates Qi on the Chong Mai
GB 26	Especially useful at ovulation through its influence on the Dai Mai ensuring the fallopian tubes are not obstructed by excess secretions
SP 5	Helpful if indications of obstruction of the fallopian tubes by excess secretions. Calms the Mind.
SP 8, SP 10, ST 29, Liv 8, BL 17 (Diaphragm Shu), BL 32	Invigorate Blood. Treat painful ovulation.
Kid 13, Kid 14, SP 13, ST 28, ST 29, Zi Gong	Regulate Qi in the ovaries & fallopian tubes
ST 30	Moves & supplements Blood. Regulates Qi. Harmonizes the Lower Burner.
Kid 5 & Kid 8	Promote ovulation by regulating Qi & Blood in Chong & Ren Mai
Kid 12, Kid 13	Tonify Kidneys & harmonize the Ren & Chong Channels. Kid 13 tonifies Jing.
Liv 3 & Liv 5	Regulate Liver Qi in the abdomen. Invigorate Blood. Drain Damp Heat from the Lower Burner. Regulate menstruation & treat dysmenorrhea caused by Liver Qi stagnation.
SP 6	Promotes Blood circulation & action of the Spleen as an intermediary between the Heart & Kidneys via the Bao Vessel and Bao Channel.

HT 5 & PC 5	Calm the Spirit & influence the Bao Vessel
PC 4	Regulates the Heart. Clears Blood Heat which may display as signs of mid-cycle spotting
Ren 4 (Uterine Point)	Tonifies & moves Blood. Warms the Uterus. Supplements the Kidneys Yin & Yang. Nourishes Jing. Opens Chong & Ren.
Du 4	Tonifies Kidney Yang. Resolves interior Cold.
Liv 2, Liv 3, Liv 14	Move Liver Qi. Treat sore breasts & irritability at ovulation.
Ren 3, Ren 12, SP 6, SP 9, Kid 7, BL 22 (San Jiao Shu), BL 28, St 40 plus ear points	Resolve Dampness & Phlegm accumulation that can lead to PCOS or fallopian tube obstruction
Kid 4, HT 7 & PC 6, Yin Tang	Calm the Shen. Regulates Bao Vessel

*Do not open the Ren & Penetrating vessels after ovulation as it could cause a miscarriage. The energy is already built up and will naturally release with a normal period.

For women who have problems with ovulation or experience a late cycle, use electro stimulation on a high pulse width with a patterning system for about 15 min. Do not use electro stim after ovulation.

With the patient in sidling position attach the positive leads to **Ren 4 (Uterus)** or **St 28 (Ovaries)** and the negative leads to Bladder points local to the ASIS (Anterior Superior Iliac Spine) such as **BL 32.** The idea is not the exactitude of the points but getting the electrical current thought the body. Blocked tubes may not respond.

Phase 4: Luteal or Pre-Menstrual Phase (Day 15 to 28)

According to Jane Lyttleton, Dip TCM and author of Treatment of Infertility with Chinese Medicine, the fundamental treatment approach in the Luteal Phase is to maintain high levels of Yang built on a solid Yin foundation established in the previous two weeks of the menstrual cycle.

Lyttleton added that boosting Yang by supplementing Yin is the most effective method of promoting implantation, nourishing the embryo and ensuring its survival.

Strong Kidney Yang helps maintain high progesterone levels which warm the Uterus and allow its walls to press inwards holding the embryo firmly in place as it burrows into the endometrium.

Three strategies can be used to boost Kidney Yang:
- Supplement Yin
- Promote Qi which is part of Yang
- Nourish Blood

When supplementing Yin in the days after ovulation the focus of treatment moves from the Chong Mai to the Ren Mai. Women with Kidney Yin Deficiency often suffer from late or irregular ovulation. The egg may be of poor quality or the Corpus Luteum may function poorly secreting inadequate levels of progesterone hindering implantation. Progesterone maintains the thick endometrial lining.

In the first week of the Luteal Phase acupuncture points that strengthen Qi help ensure the free passage of the embryo in the proximal part of the fallopian tube. Mild regulation of Blood during implantation encourages microcirculation in the endometrium and helps to calm the Mind. Once implantation has occurred avoid using herbs or acupuncture to move Blood.

The instability of Heart and Liver Qi can also hinder implantation. Premenopausal Syndrome (PMS), which often disrupts this phase, represents Liver Qi Stagnation. Breast tenderness indicates Liver Qi and Blood problems.

In ancient China PMS was called Pre-Menstrual Tension. TCM moves the Qi and Blood to release tension, calm the Mind and facilitate implantation.

Needling lower abdomen and Spleen Points is generally avoided in the week immediately before the period.

Problems Encountered During the Luteal Phase

Symptoms	Indications
Uterine lining out of sync with the day of the cycle	Kidney Yang Deficiency, Cold Uterus, Blood Stasis
Short Phase	Excess Heat, Kidney Yin Deficiency, Liver Qi Stagnation
Erratic, low & high temperatures, fatigue, inadequate luteal phase	Qi or Yang Deficiency with Liver Qi Stagnation, Spleen Qi or Kidney Yang Deficiency
Low Temperatures	Kidney Yang Deficiency
Erratically high temperatures with emotional symptoms	Spirit Disharmony. Liver & Heart Fire
Sawtooth or saddle erratic pattern	Liver & Heart Qi unstable. Kidney Yang Deficiency
Biphasic step form, slow-rising BBT during shortened Luteal Phase	Liver Qi Stagnation with Excess Heat
Slow-rise biphasic, stepwise formation	Qi Stagnation caused by Blood Stasis or Kidney Yang Deficiency
Early Decline or Luteal Phase Defect	A short or ineffective luteal phase from Kidney Yang or Spleen Qi Deficiency
PMS	Liver Qi Stagnation & Blood Stasis
Premenstrual Spotting	Qi Deficiency, Blood Stasis or pathological Heat

Several signs may point to a Luteal Phase Defect such as a shortened phase that is less than 12 days, spotting before menstruation, menopausal symptoms, or low progesterone levels midway through the luteal phase as often indicated by a slow or low rise in body temperature after ovulation.

On occasion Luteal Phase Defects result from the endometrial lining being out of sync with the release of the fertilised egg. It must be ready to receive the fertilized egg four to eight days after ovulation. Treatment for a Luteal Phase Defect focuses on supplementing Spleen Qi or Kidney Yang to raise the body's production of and response to progesterone.

In the Luteal Phase, it is appropriate to continue supporting Yin and Blood, while tonifying Yang, moving Qi and Blood to help expel Cold and warm the Uterus, resolving Dampness and normalizing Liver Qi.

Points	Effect
Kid 3, Kid 6, Kid 10, SP 6, BL 23	Encourage the development of Kidney Yang by invigorating Kidney Yin. SP 6 is the great Yin nourishing point. BL 23 nourishes Blood & tonifies Yuan & Jing Qi.
Ren 4, Kid 3, ST 36, Du 4	Tonify Kidney Yin & Yang. Ren 4 invigorates Qi & Blood in the Heart, Lungs, Kidneys, Liver & Spleen. ST 36 strengthens Qi & Blood of whole body & raises Yang.
Kid 7	Main point for tonifying Kidney Yang. Also treats dampness in the lower body & scarred fallopian tubes.
Ren 5	Regulates Qi in the Ren Mai & Uterus. Maintains good flexibility in the uterine walls (Needle only in first week after ovulation)
Ren 6	Tonifies the Kidneys & original Qi. Invigorates & regulates Blood.
Ren 7	Regulates the Ren & Chong & facilities the move from Chong to Ren (Needle just after ovulation)

ST 30 & Kid 14	Eliminate stagnation in the Penetrating Vessel
Ren 6, Ren 12, SP 6, ST 36, ST 25, BL 20	Strengthen Qi & Blood by invigorating the Spleen & Stomach
Kid 5	Enhances Blood formation via Kidney Yang
Liv 3, Liv 8, Liv 14, GB 34	Move Liver Qi & remove stagnation. Liv 8 nourishes Blood.
SP 10, BL 17	Move & cool the Blood. Directly influence Blood formation.
SP 10	Important point in treating menstrual disorders involving Blood Stasis. Resolves abdominal masses. Helps prevent clotting.
ST 28, ST 29, Liv 5, Liv 8, SP 6, SP 8, Kid 4, Kid 5	Treat Blood Stasis. SP 8 resolves Blood Stasis in the Uterus.
ST 29 with Moxa	Encourages the transport of the egg/embryo in the fallopian tube in the early part of the Luteal Phase
Liv 2, Liv 3, Liv 4, Liv 5, Liv 8, Liv 9, Liv 11, PC 5, PC 6, PC 7, Ren 3	Treat Liver & Heart Qi Stagnation. Liv 3 nourishes Liver Blood & Liver Yin. Liv 11 regulates Liver Qi in the Uterus.
Kid 7, ST 36, Ren 6, Du 4, BL 23, BL 52	Treat Luteal Phase Defect (Kidney Yang & Spleen Qi Deficiency)
Liv 2, LI 11, SP 10, BL 40	Clear excess Heat. LI 11, SP 10 & BL 40 cool the Blood.
St 30	Disperses Cold & stagnation in the pelvis.
SP 3, SP 6, SP 9, ST 40, Kid 3, ST 36, BL 20 (Spleen)	Resolve dampness & phlegm. Periods may be scanty as Uterus is congested & damp.

Ren 5 (SJ Mu), Ren 9 (Water Separation), ST 28 (Water Passage), BL 22 (SJ Shu)	Promote fluid transformation. **Ren 5** resolves dampness & phlegm in the Uterus. Moves Qi.
Kid 8	Drains damp Heat from Lower Jiao
Zi Gong	Brings Qi & Blood to the Uterus.
HT 7, Yin Tang, BL 42, Ren 15 Ear Shen Men	Spirit calming points (Shallow needling on Ren 15)
SP 4 & PC 6 - Chong Mai with Moxa on Ren 4	Apply before the arrival of menses with no signs of pregnancy to treat painful periods from Cold in the Uterus. Do not apply heat to the lower abdomen after ovulation.
GB 41 & SJ 5 - Dai Mai	Apply before menses with no signs of pregnancy to clear obstructions in the Uterus & blocked fallopian tubes, ovarian cysts & painful periods.

Normally treatment to strongly move Blood must wait for the first signs of a period or for a drop in the BBT. If there are no signs of pregnancy increased menstrual flow can be encouraged up to one week before the arrival of menses.

Points to Regulated the Hypothalamic-Pituitary-Ovarian Axis
- SP 4 & PC 6 - Penetrating Vessel
- LU 7 & KID 6 - Conception Vessel
- BL 62 & SI 3 - Governing Vessel
Plus SP 6, Ren 3, Ren 4 & Zi Gong

Auricular Therapy
Activate points in the triangular fossa that stimulate the Uterus and fallopian tubes, calm the spirit, regulate the sympathetic nervous system, and reduce overall tension and Blood pressure. Activate points in the intertragic notch that stimulate the endocrine and ovaries.

Scalp Acupuncture
The Epang scalp reproductive points regulate the reproductive and pelvic function including dysmenorrhea. They reinforce the Kidneys, regulate menstruation and treat acute urinary dysfunction.

Deficient & Excess Types of Infertility

Deficient Types of Infertility

1. Kidney Qi, Yin and Yang Deficiency
2. Blood Deficiency
3. Heart Qi & Yang Deficiency

Excess Types of Infertility

1. Blood Stasis
2. Stagnation of Cold in the Uterus
3. Dampness in the Lower Jiao
4. Blood Heat
5. Qi Stagnation
6. Liver Qi Stagnation
7. Heart Qi Not Descending or Heart Fire

Most patients manifest mixed patterns (combinations of 2 or 3, or more). Therefore, the treatment, including the selection of acupoints, needs to be modified accordingly.

Deficient Types of Infertility

1. Kidney Qi, Yin and Yang Deficiency
2. Blood Deficiency
3. Heart Qi & Yang Deficiency

1. Kidney Qi Deficiency

Kidney Qi deficiency is one of the most common causes of infertility. In Chinese medicine, the Kidney system provides the energy required for reproduction.

If this energy is deficient either from overwork, a weak constitution, excessive sex or other health issues, it may lead to a deficiency of the Conception and Penetrating Vessels which are central to providing the Uterus with Tian Gui (Menstrual Blood).

The literal translation of Tian Gui is "heavenly water," and heavenly water mixed with sperm yields pregnancy. The weakening of the menstrual Blood may cause the Uterus to become malnourished so that it cannot collect sperm and promote conception.

General Signs & Symptoms
- General weakness and fatigue
- Lower Back Pain
- Loose stools
- Weak voice/reluctance to speak
- Loss of sexual energy or desire
- Prolonged cycle
- Scanty flow
- Dizziness
- Frequent urination
- Long term infertility

Pulse: Weak or fine
Tongue: Overall pale and not well defined

Possible Treatment Points

Lu 7 Right & **Kid 6** Left - Opens the Ren Channel which has domain over hormones.
Kid 13 - Nourish the Penetrating Channel (Chong Mai). Strengthens the Kidney & Uterus
Kid 3, BL 23 (L2), BL 52 (L2) - Tonifies the Kidney & nourishes Essence
Ren 4, ST 28 (Bilateral) - Nourishes Blood, ovaries and Uterus
Ren 7 - Regulates the Uterus. Nourishes Yin.
St 36 & Sp 6 (CI Pregnancy) - Nourishes Blood
BL 17 (T7) with Moxa (Sea of Blood Point – Diaphragm Shu) Nourishes Essence, strengthens the Uterus & promotes fertility.

Plus additional points
SP 4 & PC 6 – Opens Penetrating Vessel - Menstruation must be normalized first.
Kid I2 – Tonifies Kidneys & Yuan Qi. Harmonizes Ren & Chong Vessels
Ren 6 – Tonifies Original Qi

There are two types of Kidney Deficiency, Kidney Yin and Kidney Yang Deficiency:

1.1   Kidney Yin Deficiency

Yin Deficiency = Dry mucus membranes
Kidney Yin Deficiency = Dry vagina
Liver Yin Deficiency = Dry eyes
Lung Yin Deficiency = Dry nose
Stomach Yin Deficiency = Dry mouth

Signs & Symptoms
- Long-term infertility
- Short menstrual cycle
- Scanty pale menstrual discharge
- Lack of menstruation
- Constipation
- Mallor flush
- Night sweats
- Insomnia
- Dry throat
- Heat in the palms, soles, and chest
- Irritability
- Aversion to heat or sensations of heat in the afternoon or evening
- Difficulty sleeping
- Dizziness
- Possible palpitations
- Hyperactive sex drive
- Weakness in the lower back and knees
- Tinnitus

In men, symptoms may include decreased ability to control ejaculation or abnormally protracted erections.

Tongue: Red with a scanty or no coat, peeled and dry
Pulse: Floating, fine, thin, empty or rapid
Tx: Nourish Kidney Yin and Kidney Essence

Possible Treatment Points
LU 7 (Right) & **Kid 6** (Left) – Opens Ren Mai. Nourishes Kidney Yin.
Ren 4, Ren 7, Kid 13 – Nourish Kidney Essence. Strengthens the Ren & Penetrating Channels
Kid 3, Kid 6, Kid 10, SP 6 - Nourish Kidney Yin
BL 23 (Kidney Shu) - Supports Kidneys & Essence
BL 52 - Strengthens willpower. Supports Kidneys & Essence.

Reinforcing method. Generally, no moxa unless the tongue is not red or only slightly red with a very fine pulse. A small amount of moxa on Kid 3 helps increase the tonification effect.

1.2 Kidney Yang Deficiency

Signs & Symptoms
- Late periods with pale menstrual discharge
- Irregular menstruation with scanty pinkish Blood
- Lack of menstruation
- Leucorrhea
- Diarrhea with periods or loose stools
- Odema
- Chills
- Aversion to cold
- Pale complexion
- Fatigue
- Weak lower back and knees
- Frequent urination with profuse clear urine
- Low sex drive
- Dizziness
- Depression

In men, symptoms may also include impotence and sensations of cold in the scrotum.

Tongue: Pale, swollen, wet, with thin white coat
Pulse: Deep, slow, thin, particularly weak in the Kidney position
Tx: Tonify Kidney Yang, Warm the Gate of vitality, Strengthen the Uterus

Possible Treatment Points (Reinforcing Method)
LU 7 (Right) & **Kid 6** (Left) - Opens the Ren Mai
Lu 7 & **SP 4** - Regulates & nourishes Ren & Chong, & normalises irregular menstruation.
BL 23 (Kidney Shu) - Supports Kidneys & Essence
BL 52 - Tonify psycho-emotional aspects of the Kidneys. Supports Kidneys & Essence
Ren 4, Ren 8, Du 4 with Moxa or FIL- Tonify Yang. Strengthens the Uterus. Warms the Gate of Vitality

ST 36 - Tonifies Original Qi. Nourishes Blood.
Kid 3 & Kid 7 - Strengthen Kidney Yang
Kid 13 - Important point for infertility. Nourishes the Chong Mai & Kidneys. Strengthens the Uterus.
Kid 2 - Fire point, usually used to disperse empty fire rising causing sore throat. Here it is used with moxa to strengthen & warm the Uterus
SJ 17 - If dizziness &/or tinnitus
Kid 10 - If weak back &/or knees
BL 32 - Tonifies the Kidneys

1.3 Kidney Yin & Yang Deficiency

Kidney Qi Deficiency in women over 40 years old is nearly always a deficiency of both Yin and Yang with a predominance of either Yin or Yang Deficiency. This pathology accounts for many contradictory symptoms of simultaneous Heat and Cold. It is not Full or Empty Heat because of the presence of Cold symptoms such as cold feet and a Pale tongue.

Signs & Symptoms
- Heavy periods
- Early and scanty periods if Yin Deficiency predominates
- Late periods if Yang Deficiency predominates
- Hot flashes with Cold hands & feet
- Frequent, pale urination if Yang deficiency predominates
- Frequent urination if Yin Deficiency predominates
- Feels chilled in general but with hot flashes or hot feet
- Feeling of Heat with night sweats but cold feet
- Dry throat
- Dizziness
- Backache
- Possibly low libido

Tongue: Pale or red (pale more Yang Deficiency and red more Yin Deficiency)
Pulse: Floating, empty or thin, rapid (if Yin Deficient) or deep, weak (if Yang Deficient)
Tx: Tonify Kidneys, Tonify Yin, Gently Tonify Yang

Possible Treatment Points
Lu 7 & Kid 6 – Opens Ren Mai. Strengthens the Uterus & nourishes Kidney Yin.

Kid 3 – Tonifies Jing & Kidney Yin
HT 6 & Kid 7 – Night sweats. Clears Empty Heat.
Ren 4 – Tonifies Jing, & Kidney Yin & Yang. Calms the Mind.
SP 6 - Tonifies Yin, nourishes, harmonizes & invigorates Blood
BL 23 (Kidney Shu) – Tonifies Yang & Original Qi
BL 52 - Supports BL 23, and can affect Yang as well as emotions.

Contradictory symptoms of Heat and Cold may be the result of Rebellious Qi of the Chong Mai, which is caused by a Deficiency of Qi in the Lower Dantian. In this pathology the Qi of the Chong Mai does not flow down to the feet, so they feel cold. The Qi rebels upwards creating a feeling of heat in the face. Other signs and symptoms are present in each of the three Dantians.

Yin Fire can also cause contradictory symptoms. According to Giovanni Maciocia, Yin Fire is neither Full Heat nor Empty Heat but simply a different kind of Heat that derives from a deficiency of the Yuan Qi.

Suspect Yin Fire whenever there is:
- Deficiency of the Yuan Qi manifesting with great tiredness
- Heat above with a red face, thirst, or mouth ulcers
- Cold symptoms with a feeling Cold in general
- Pale tongue

Blood Deficiency leading to Empty Heat especially in women may also lead to contradictory symptoms of Heat and Cold.

Kidney Essence Deficiency in women is indicated by empty follicles, low ovarian reserve at a young age (under the age of 30), dizziness, hair loss, blurred vision, and infertility. In men, it is often represented by azoospermia or the absence of motile sperm in the semen in the absence of anatomical anomalies.

2. Blood Deficiency

Blood is the material basis for conception. It is derived mostly from the Gu Qi (food qi) produced by the Spleen. When an individual has a constitutional weakness or dysfunction in the Spleen and Stomach, Blood production is affected. As a result, the extra meridians become deficient or dysfunctional and the Uterus is not nourished making it impossible for a woman to conceive.

The Liver stores the Blood and provides Blood to the Uterus in close coordination with the Chong Mai. Women are particularly prone to Blood Deficiency due to loss of Blood during the menses as well as from diet, overwork, and emotional stress.

Blood Deficiency originating from Liver and Spleen Deficiency is ordinary Blood and not Tian Gui. Tian Gui which is the source of menstrual Blood or menstrual water, originates from the Kidneys.

Therefore, in gynecological problems from Blood Deficiency tonify the Liver and Kidney Yang Qi which will strengthen Jing. The Spleen may also be tonified to indirectly help the production of Tian Gui.

Signs & Symptoms
- Short or delayed menstruation with scanty, pinkish flow
- Pale Blood (Almost brown as bleeding so slow the Blood dries up)
- Weakness of the body
- Dry skin and/or hair
- Pale complexion
- Fatigue
- Dizziness
- Depression
- Tingling
- Blurred vision
- Brittle nails
- Cramps
- May also have palpitations and/or insomnia if Heart Blood is deficient
Tongue: Pale, thin & slightly dry, possibly swollen due to the presence of Dampness & Phlegm
Pulse: Deep, choppy, fine, weak
Tx: Nourish Blood and Essence, Strengthen Liver and Kidneys

Treatment of Blood deficiency depends on two factors:
- Which organ is affected
- Whether it is a deficiency of so-called ordinary Blood or of Tian Gui.

The following suggested points are for treating gynecological conditions.

Possible Treatment Points (Reinforcing Method – Moxa Applicable)
SP 4 (Right) & **PC 6** (Left) - Opens & regulates the Penetrating Vessel
LU 7 (Right) & **Kid 6** (Left) - Opens the Ren Channel
Ren 4 - Tonify Yin & Blood. Strengthens the Uterus.
Liv 8 - Nourishes Blood. Sedates the Liver. Nourishes the Kidneys
ST 36 & SP 6 - Nourishes Blood & Qi
Kid 3 - Nourishes Essence. Tonifies Kidney Yin.
Kid 13 - Nourishes the Penetrating Vessel, the Kidneys & strengthens
the Uterus. Harmonizes the Ren & Chong Vessels.
Zi Gong (3 cun lateral to Ren 3) – Nourishes Essence & fertility. Brings
Qi & Blood to the Uterus.
BL 11 (Sea of Blood Point) - Tonifies & Nourishes Blood
BL 17 (Diaphragm Shu & Sea of Blood Point - **Direct Moxa**) –
Nourishes Blood & Essence. Strengthens the Uterus.
BL 18 (Liver Shu) - Sedates the Liver & nourishes Liver Blood
BL 20 (Spleen Shu) - Transforms Dampness & nourishes Blood
BL 23 (Kidney Shu) - Nourishes Blood & Tonifies Jing & Yuan Qi
SP 10 - If signs of hot Blood
HT 7 - If insomnia/palpitations
GV 20 - If dizziness

Pathologies deriving from Liver Blood Deficiency

- Liver Qi Stagnation	- Kidney Yang or Yin Deficiency
- Liver Blood Stasis	- Qi Deficiency
- Liver Yang Rising	- Cold in the Uterus
- Heart Blood Deficiency	- Cold Limbs
- Empty Heat	- Wind Heat (Skin)

3. Heart Qi & Yang Deficiency

In general deficiencies of Heart Qi and Yang involve more physical
symptoms, while Heart Blood and Yin Deficiency involve more
mental-emotional disturbances, and somewhat fewer physical
symptoms.

This is because the Qi and Yang move the Blood (active function of
circulation), while the Blood and Yin house the mental consciousness.
Heart Qi and Heart Yang are closely related, Heart Yang being a
broader, more inclusive category.

When it is necessary to nourish Blood in gynecological problems, one possibility is to nourish Heart Blood with points such as HE 7 and BL 15 (Heart Shu). HE 5 can be used for heavy periods or flooding and trickling, especially in combination with Liv 2 and SP 6

There are three primary causes of Heart Qi and Heart Yang deficiency:

1) Prolonged illness, surgery, acute or chronic bleeding
2) Overwork, excessive exercise or sex
3) Emotional problems: especially sadness, melancholy, anger, fright, worry or over-thinking

While sadness relates to the Lungs in the 5 Element Theory, sadness affects the Heart Qi because the Heart and Lungs are closely related and mutually assist each other. Sadness weakens Lung Qi which can cause Heart Qi to become deficient.

Prolonged sadness and Deficient Qi can also lead to Stagnation of Qi, which can lead to Heart Fire. While Anger affects the Liver directly, it affects the Heart indirectly. Anger causes Liver Yang to rise, which can eventually be transmitted to the Heart, causing Heart Fire.

Blood Loss or severe bleeding affecting the Heart

Severe Blood loss from a hemorrhage or long-term illness can deplete Heart Blood (Heart rules Blood), and this can lead to Heart Qi Deficiency

3.1. Heart Qi Deficiency

Signs & Symptoms

The signs include not only general Qi Deficiency signs, but signs specific to Heart Qi Deficiency, like palpitations.

- Palpitations (a common symptom in all Heart deficiencies due to Heart Qi deficiency)
- Fatigue
- Lethargy (Worse with exercise)
- Shortness of breath (worse with activity); may also be hurried breathing
- Weak voice

- Pale, bright face
- Spontaneous, daytime perspiration
- May be disturbances of Blood circulation
- Spirits may be "darkened" or "tired"

Tongue: Normal color. In more severe cases, pale, often enlarged with scallops. Thin, white coating.

Pulse: Thready and feeble or weak, or irregular (choppy, knotted or intermittent)

Tx: Tonify Heart Qi

Possible Acupuncture Points

HT 5 - Tonifies Heart Qi

PC 6 - Tonifies Heart Qi. Calms the Mind

BL 15 (Heart Shu Point) - With moxa. Warms & tonifies Heart Yang

REN 17 - With Moxa. Influential Point of Qi. Warms & tonifies Heart Yang

REN 6 - With Moxa. Warm & tonify Yang of the whole body. Use if Heart Yang Deficiency is due to Kidney Yang Deficiency

3.2 Heart Yang Deficiency

Because the Kidneys are the source of Yang for all the internal organs, chronic Kidney Yang Deficiency can lead to Heart Yang Deficiency.

All the above symptoms (under Heart Qi Deficiency), with greater severity, plus **signs and symptoms of Cold**:

- Sensation of cold, person feels chilled inside
- Cold limbs and hands
- Dusky, dark (or purplish) complexion. Sometimes it is bright pale.
- Darkish (cyanotic or purplish) lips
- Profuse, spontaneous perspiration
- Swelling (edema), especially in the upper body
- Shortness of breath with asthmatic breathing
- May be stuffiness or pain in the chest or precordial region (Over the Heart or Stomach) due to Cold. (In severe cases of pain Blood stasis is also indicated.)

Tongue: Like Heart Qi deficiency, except more swollen and moist. Like the complexion, it may be dark (dusky).

Pulse: Same as Heart Qi Deficiency but may also be slow or knotted in severe cases.

Tx: Tonify and warm Heart Yang

Possible Acupuncture Points

HT 5 - Tonifies Heart Qi

PC 6 - Tonifies Heart Qi. Calms the Mind

BL 15 (Heart Shu Point) - With moxa. Warms & Tonifies Heart Yang

REN 17 (Pericardium Mu Point) - With Moxa. Influential Point of Qi. Warms & tonifies Heart Yang

REN 6 - With Moxa. Warm & tonify Yang of the whole body. Use if Heart Yang Deficiency is due to Kidney Yang Deficiency

DU 14 - With Moxa. Tonify Heart Yang

Method: Tonify all Points. Moxa used where applicable.

Excess Types of Infertility

1. Blood Stasis
2. Stagnation of Cold in the Uterus
3. Dampness in the Lower Jiao
4. Blood Heat
5. Qi Stagnation
6. Liver Qi Stagnation
7. Heart Qi Not Descending or Heart Fire

1. Blood Stasis

There are two types of Blood Stasis in the body:

- Blood that has leaked from the vessels and is lodged in the tissues due to physical trauma.
- Blood that has stagnated in the meridians and organs such as the Uterus.

Major Causes of Blood Stasis in the Uterus

- Qi Stagnation
- Qi and Blood Deficiency
- Hemorrhage causing pooling & stagnation of extravasated Blood
- Invasion of Cold or Heat
- Emotional Trauma
- Long term illness
- Damage to the Uterus during a previous delivery
- Engaging In sex during menses
- Long term use of an Intrauterine Device

Accumulation of Phlegm can be an aggravating factor.

There are four stages in the evolution of Blood Stasis moving from a mild to a more severe condition:
- Painful periods, dark Blood with clots with a normal tongue
- Purple sublingual veins
- Purple sides of tongue
- Whole tongue purple (Very advanced stage)

Blood Stasis is a major pathology in gynecology and left untreated can lead to serious disease such as endometriosis, cervical cancer, uterine cancer, POS, and myomas. Always suspect Blood Stasis in chronic complicated gynecological conditions.

Blood Stasis can cause heavy menstrual bleeding as new Blood, blocked by Stagnant Liver Blood, is forced out of the Uterus. This type of bleeding is characterized by severe fixed pain, and discharge of dark or clotted Blood.

Blood Stasis presents in combination with other pathogenic factors such as:

- **Qi Stagnation**: Symptoms of stuffiness in the chest, indigestion, swollen mass in the abdomen with stabbing pain, irregular menstruation, distention in the breast, purple tongue with bruising, and sluggish pulse.

- **Blood Deficiency:** Symptoms of dizziness, palpitations, insomnia, and a tongue that is pale rather than purple. Indicative of Blood Stasis with underlying Blood Deficiency. The body does not have enough Blood to properly circulate, so the Blood becomes sluggish and stagnates.

- **Cold:** Symptoms of cold limbs made better upon warming. Called pathogenic cold invading the meridians causing Blood Stasis. This can also show up as painful menstrual period, delayed menstruation with dark purple clots, pale tongue, and a pulse that feels deep and slow. In this case the cold has caused the Blood to congeal and become sluggish. This leads to pain and the other symptoms mentioned above.

- **Blood Heat:** Blood Heat is the most common pattern of uterine bleeding. Heat from the Liver or the Heart can enter the Blood causing reckless movement of Blood leading to Uterine bleeding or can also dry the Blood leading to amenorrhea.

Blood Heat can also arise from chronic Blood Stasis. Symptoms of heat are present such as a red dry tongue and rapid pulse.

Signs & Symptoms
- Heavy menstrual bleeding
- Pain in the pre-menstrual phase relieved by the onset of menses
- Painful irregular periods (Periods stopping and starting)
- Dark Menstrual Blood
- Large, dark clots
- Abdominal masses such as cysts, endometriosis or myomas
- Fixed masses on the surface of the body
- Stabbing pain worse with pressure that is fixed, stabbing, severe
- Dark complexion
- Rough scaly dry skin
- Dry hair
- Purple lips and finger nails
- Irritability
- Manic behavior
- Abdominal pain during menses
- Unsettled Mind leading to insomnia, excessive dreaming, mental restlessness & agitation.

Expect hot flashes in women experiencing a long period of perimenopause. In men, there may be an enlargement of the veins of the scrotum or a history of hernia.

Tongue: Purple (Reddish Purple with Heat; More common Bluish Purple with Cold) Sometimes only the sides of the tongue are Purple when there is Blood Stasis in the Uterus.
Pulse: Wiry, Firm or possibly Choppy.
Tx: Depending on the root cause remove Blood Stasis by moving Qi, expelling Cold, clearing Heat or resolving Phlegm. Invigorate Blood.

Possible Treatment Points (Reducing or Even Method)
Sp 4 (Right) & **PC 6** (Left) – Opens & regulates the Penetrating Vessel. Moves Blood.
LU 7 (Right) & **Kid 6** (Left) – Opens the Ren Channel
Liv 3 & **GB 34** – Moves Liver Qi. Removes stagnation
BL 17 (Sea of Blood Point) – Cools & nourishes Blood
SP 10, SP 6 & PC 6 – Tonifies & cools Blood. Removes Stasis.
Ren 4 – Supports the Uterus and Blood. Removes stagnation.

Ren 6 & SJ 6 – Strongly tonifies & moves Qi
ST 29 & Kid 14 – Eliminates stagnation in the Penetrating Vessel & moves Qi & Blood
ST 36 – Nourishes Blood. Tonifies Original Qi.
BL 40 – Invigorates the Blood. Clears Heat.

2. Stagnation of Cold in the Uterus (Excess Yin)

Cold obstructs the Uterus, therefore Liver Blood cannot be stored properly in the Uterus which may lead to Blood Deficiency. Therefore, Cold and Blood Deficiency often coexist.

Cold in the Uterus also leads to Qi Stagnation and Blood Stasis which can cause dysmenorrhea (painful periods), amenorrhea (absence of periods), prolonged menstruation and the accumulation of abdominal masses. In less severe cases the length of the menstrual cycle may not be affected.

Cold in the Uterus may come from the exterior via the female reproductive organs, from Cold stagnating in the Liver channel, or from Kidney Yang Deficiency. During puberty, girls are especially susceptible to Cold and Dampness. This can lead to cold obstructions in the Uterus, Ren and Penetrating channels.

Chronic exposure to cold and damp food and environments during menstruation can also disrupt the Uterus, and lead to the accumulation of Cold or Damp. Moxa or Far Infrared Light must always be used in this treatment to expel Cold. The menstrual Blood must be warmed to dispel Blood Stasis.

The Yang Qi is predominant after ovulation, creating movement and warming the Uterus. Therefore, the best time to expel stagnation from the Uterus is during the Luteal and Menstrual Phases, unless there is excessive bleeding during menses at which time it is advisable not to intensify the downward movement of Blood.

If the patient is actively trying to get pregnant do not try to expel pathogenic factors from the Uterus during the Ovulation Phase, and into the beginning of the Luteal Phase. Only resume treatment to remove stagnation when it is determined there is no pregnancy. To avoid increasing temperature of the Uterus during implantation of an embryo, do not apply Heat to the Lower Abdomen after ovulation.

Signs & Symptoms
- Normal or delayed menstruation with dark diluted flow
- Pain and/or coldness of the lower abdomen which improves with the application of heat
- Abdominal cramps relieved by Heat
- Painful periods especially in young girls and young women
- Small dark clots
- Pale face
- Aversion to cold
- Generally cold during menses
- May have weak back/knees and/or profuse clear urination

Tongue: Pale or Bluish Purple with a thick white coating
Pulse: Choppy & Slow or Tight & Slow
Tx: Expel Cold. Warm and tonify Kidney Yang and the Uterus.

Possible Acupuncture Points (Reinforcing Method with Moxa)
SP 4 (Right) & **PC 6** (Left) – Opens the Chong or Penetrating Vessel. Moves Blood.
GB 41 (Left) & **SJ 5** (Right) – Regulates the Girdle Vessel or Dai Mai. Releases blockages in Lower Jiao.
Ren 2 - Cold Uterus
Ren 4 with Moxa – Strengthens the Kidneys. Fortifies original Qi. Warms the Uterus. Reduces Abdominal Pain.
Ren 6 - Tonifies & warms the Lower Burner
DU 4 with Moxa – Tonifies Kidney Yang. Expels Cold. Strengthens Jing & the Gate of Vitality.
Kid 3 & **Kid 7** – Strengthens Kidney Yang
BL 23 (Kidney Shu) – Warms the Uterus. Tonifies Jing & Kidney Yang.
ST 29 -Warms the Lower Jiao. Invigorates Blood & regulates menstruation
ST 36 – Tonifies Original Qi. Nourishes & invigorates Blood. (Reinforcing Method).
SP 8 – Regulates menstruation & invigorates Blood.
Liv 3 & **SP 6** – Moves Qi & Blood in the Uterus. Activates the energy of the Chong Mai.

3. Dampness in the Lower Jiao

Improper dietary habits or Yang Deficiency in the Kidney and Spleen lead to a dysfunction in the water metabolism which can cause accumulation of Dampness and Phlegm.

When the body has too much Dampness and Phlegm, the movement of Blood and Qi is disturbed and the meridians around the Uterus are obstructed resulting in irregular menses and conception problems. The congenital essence from both sexes will have difficulty joining in the embryo.

Signs & Symptoms
- Long-term infertility
- Large amount of vaginal discharge with no menses
- Prolonged menstrual cycle
- Irregular periods
- Pain at ovulation
- Vaginal discharge
- Obesity
- Sensation of bodily heaviness
- Mind not clear
- Expectoration of copious amounts of phlegm
- Possible dizziness or palpitations
- Urinary or genital issues in women.
In men, there may be an accumulation of fluid in the scrotum.

Tongue: Sticky. May have a greasy white coating
Pulse: May be slippery or slippery and wiry.
Tx: Resolve Damp. Remove obstructions in Penetrating & Ren vessels.

Possible Acupuncture Points (Reducing or even method. No moxa)
LU 7 (Right) & **Kid 6** (Left) - Opens the Ren Channel
Ren 3 & **Zi Gong** (3 cun lateral to Ren 3) - Strengthens the Uterus. Removes dampness.
SP 3, SP 6, SP 9, ST 40 - Resolves Dampness
ST 30 & KID 14 – Eliminates stagnation in the Penetrating vessel.
REN 9 - Expels Dampness. Tonifies the Spleen. Regulates Water Passages.
REN 12 - Expels Dampness. Tonifies the Spleen
ST 36 - Expels Dampness. Tonifies the Spleen

Liv 5 – Major Point for vaginal Infections. Treats Damp Heat, genital pain & irregular menses

BL 22 (San Jiao Shu) – Drains Damp Heat from the Lower Burner. Tonifies the Spleen.

SJ 4 & BL 64 – Needled together these points move Qi in the San Jiao (Triple Burner) & open the water passages.

The Dai Mai or Girdling Vessel is used to treat dampness in the genital region and Lower Burner, irregular periods, abdominal pain from painful periods (dysmenorrhoea), blocked fallopian tubes and ovarian cysts.

The Kidney's functions of storing essence and lowering and holding Qi, the Spleen's function of raising Qi, and the Liver's function of smoothing the flow of Qi all rely on the proper functioning of the Dai Mai which encircles the body at the waist. Impairment of the Girdling Vessel can weaken the Spleen contributing to Dampness which may infuse downwards and cause excessive vaginal discharge. Deficiency of the Girdling vessel may also result in the sinking of Spleen Qi, which can induce a prolapse of the Uterus.

GB 41 (Right) & **SJ 5** (Left) - Regulates the Girdling Vessel. Drains Damp Heat in the Lower Burner.

GB 26 - Connects with the Dai Mai. Regulates the Uterus, drains damp Heat in the Lower Jiao, and treats leucorrhoea, a whitish or yellowish discharge of mucus from the vagina.

BL 32 - Connects with the Dai Mai. Treats pelvic area problems. Invigorates Blood. Tonifies the Kidneys.

Ren 4 - Tonifies Original Qi & Kidneys. Calms the Spirit. Regulates the Uterus & promotes fertility.

Plus Electro-Stim - Attach the positive red leads to **Ren 4 (Uterus)** or **St 28 (Ovaries)** and the negative black leads to **BL 32**.

4. Blood Heat

Blood Heat is marked by excess heat pressing the Blood out of the vessels. This condition may develop from prolonged stagnation of Liver Qi, from emotional stress and diet, or by the flaring up of the pathological Minister Fire.

Signs & Symptoms
- Short or early periods
- Heavy flow with bright-red Blood indicating full Heat
- Heavy prolonged flow with scarlet-red Blood
- 5 Palm Heat, night sweats & malar flush indicating Empty Heat
- Feeling heat during menses
- Thirst
- Mental restlessness

Tongue: Red
Pulse: Rapid and overflowing
Tx: Cool Blood, Support Yin

Possible Acupuncture Points (Reducing or Even Method – No moxa)
Sp 4 (Right) & **PC 6** (Left) - Opens & regulates the Penetrating Vessel
LU 7 (Right) & **Kid 6** (Left) - Opens the Ren Channel
LI 11, Kid 2, Liv 2, Liv 3, SP 6, SP 10, PC 3 – All points cool Blood & remove stasis.
Ren 4 - Supports the Uterus and Blood
BL 17 - (Sea of Blood Point) – Cools & nourishes Blood

5. Qi Stagnation

Qi Stagnation may affect any of the organ systems and not only the Liver. May result from physical trauma, poor diet, depression or opportunistic infections.

Signs & Symptoms
- Irregular periods
- PMS
- Painful Periods
- Breast distension
- Irritability

Tongue: Normal or red on the sides
Pulse: Wiry
Tx: Remove stagnation. Mover Liver Qi.

Possible Acupuncture Points
Sp 4 (Right) & **PC 6** (Left) – Opens & regulates the Penetrating Vessel
Liv 3, GB 34 & SJ 6 – Moves Liver Qi. Removes stagnation.
Ren 4 – Supports the Uterus & Blood

Ren 6 – Tonifies upright Qi
ST 30 & Kid 14 – Eliminates stagnation in the Penetrating Vessel

6. Liver Qi Stagnation

Liver Qi Stagnation often occurs from emotional stress driven by excessive anger, worry, shame or guilt. It manifests itself mainly in phase four of the menstrual cycle as Premenstrual Syndrome (PMS).

A major focus of infertility treatments is the regulation of the menstrual cycle and the treatment of any associated issues such as PMS or dysmenorrhea. Regulation of the Liver organ system is an important aspect of treatment as the Liver regulates the smooth flow of Qi and Blood.

After the Kidneys, the Liver exercises the greatest influence in gynecology. A Deficiency of Liver Blood and Liver Qi Stagnation are very common in women. This condition often leads to Liver Yang rising which may cause headaches before or during menses.

General Symptoms
- Irregular menstrual cycles with cramps (Early or Delayed)
- Heavy periods with dark menstrual discharge and clots
- Premenstrual tension relieved by menses
- Painful periods relieved by Heat
- Distention of the lower abdomen, epigastrium or breasts especially during the pre-menstrual phase
- Adhesions
- Obesity
- Mental restlessness

In men, symptoms may include sagging pain in the scrotum, inability to maintain an erection, and difficulty ejaculating.

Tongue: Normal or possible redness on the sides of the tongue with severe Liver Qi Stagnation.
Pulse: Wiry, choppy, rapid, slippery, tight

Possible Treatments Points
SP 4 Right **& PC 6** Left - Regulates the Penetrating Vessel
Lu 7 Right & **Kid 6** Left - Opens Ren Channel. Tonifies Yin, Uterus & Ovaries.

GB 41 Right & **SJ 5** Left - Regulates the Belt Vessel & drains Dampness. Supports the Liver's function of smoothing the flow of Qi.
Ren 2, Ren 4, Du 4 with Moxa - Local points to strengthen the Uterus
Ren 3 & Zi Gong (3 cun lateral to Ren 3) Bilateral - Strengthens Uterus & removes dampness.
St 30 & Kid 14 (Pts of intersection with Chong) - Eliminates stagnation in the Penetrating Vessel.
BL 32 - Electro stim (Black lead) & **Ren 4** (Red lead) - Blocked fallopian tubes. (**St 28** for ovaries – Red lead anterior)
Li 11, SP 10, Kid 2 & Liv 3, Sp 6 & PC 3 - Cool Blood & remove stagnation.
Liv 3, GB 34, GB 41 - Moves Liver Qi & removes stagnation
St 29 - Invigorates Blood

NOTE: PC 6 has a strong effect on moving Blood. **SP 10** is the best point to cool Blood. Not as excessive as **Liv 2.**

Auricular Therapy: Shen Men, Zero Point, Ovary Point close to ovulation.

7. Heart Qi Not Descending or Heart Fire

The Heart plays a role in the formation of menstrual Blood. It promotes the discharge of Blood at menstruation and the release of eggs at ovulation. Due to the connection via the Uterus Vessel between Heart and the Uterus, emotional issues have a direct influence on menstruation.

Pensiveness and worry agitate the Heart. The Emperor Fire fails to communicate with the Kidneys. Water and Fire do not communicate resulting in interruption of menses and infertility.

In the Five Element Theory, the Kidney water calms the Heart Fire and the Heart Fire warms the Kidney water. Healthy Kidneys play an important role in calming the Heart Fire. Communication between the Heart and Kidneys is essential for a healthy sexual, reproductive and mental-emotional life.

The strategy to treat **Heart Qi Not Descending** is to calm the Heart Fire and strengthen the Kidney Qi.

Signs & Symptoms
A condition of extreme restlessness or manic behavior indicates possible Heat in the Heart.

Other possible S/S:
- Delayed or absence of periods
- Scanty periods
- Insomnia
- Excessive dreaming
- Thirst
- Feverishness or flushed face
- Bitter taste in the mouth
- Scanty, dark urine
- Ulcers, sores of the mouth and tongue

Tongue: Red or red tipped. Crimson to scarlet. Sometimes red spots on the tongue. Often yellow fur.
Pulse: Rapid

Possible Treatment Points
Ren 4 – Tonifies Original Qi & Kidneys. Calms the Spirit. Regulates the Uterus & promotes fertility.
KID 13 – Harmonizes Ren & Chong Vessels. Lowers Lung Qi (When the Penetrating vessel is diseased there is counter-flow Qi - Classic of Difficulties)
HT 5 – Calms the Spirit. Regulates Heart Qi. Lowers Lung Qi.
Ren 14 & BL 15 – Agitated Heart
Ren 15 (Great Luo Connecting Point – Descends & disperses Qi over the abdomen) – Regulates Heart Qi. Calms the Spirit. Lowers Lung Qi & unbinds the chest.

For Rebellious Qi and Heart Fire causing breathlessness
HT 7 - Calms the Spirit. Regulates the Heart & clears the Mind
SP 9 - Treats Dampness that creates a feeling of fullness in the region below the Heart that can lead to shortness of breath or dyspnoea
BL 60 – Clears Heat. Lowers Yang.
GB 41 – Opens & releases the chest

Retroverted Uterus

Normally, the Uterus tips slightly forward towards the Stomach. Some women have a Uterus that is more vertical or tilts backwards towards the spine. This is commonly referred to as a tipped or retroverted Uterus, which affects more than 20% of women worldwide.

A retroverted Uterus can occasionally be painful or signal an underlying health disorder. Certain factors can cause a Uterus that is in a normal placement to become retroverted such as pregnancy or menopause which can weaken the ligaments that keep the Uterus in place.

Reproductive health problems such as Pelvic Inflammatory Disease and Endometriosis can cause scaring. The resulting adhesions can cause the Uterus to shift to a tilted position.

A pregnant woman with a retroverted Uterus may suffer from low back pain and constipation until the adhesions holding the Uterus to the posterior wall break free normally around 14 weeks into the pregnancy.

Possible Treatment Points
Ren 4 - Regulates the Uterus. Treats lower abdominal pain.
Ren 6 - Gynecological disorders
Ren 12 - Releases pressure in the upper abdomen.
BL 20 (T11 - Spleen Shu) – Lower back pain. Gynecological disorders. Treats pressure in the upper abdomen.
BL 23 (L2) - Gynecological disorders. Strengthens tendons. Lower back pain.
BL 32 - Gynecological disorders. Lower back pain.
KID 3 - Strengthens lower back.
SJ 4 - Relaxes rigidity in the tendons
DU 20 - Uplifts the Qi. Treats prolapses.

Ectopic Pregnancy

An ectopic pregnancy occurs when a fertilized egg implants and grows outside the main cavity of the Uterus instead of in the endometrial lining. The fertilized egg often implants in a fallopian tube but may migrate to other areas of the body such as the ovary, abdominal cavity or cervix.

Ectopic pregnancies may be caused by:

- Obstructions in the fallopian tubes cause by surgical intervention, accumulation of mucus or previous infections such as Chronic Pelvic Inflammatory Disease
- Absence of a protective lining on the outside of the fallopian tubes from low mucus production
- Thinning of the mucus on the inner walls of the fallopian tubes due to increased levels of progesterone. The lining on the inner walls of the fallopian tubes nourishes the embryo and facilitates its passage into the Uterus.

Traditional Chinese Medicine attributes ectopic pregnancies to Blood and Qi Stagnation. When congestion of Dampness and Phlegm is added to this mix it creates the ideal environment for the accumulation of excess mucus in the reproductive system which can block the movement of the fertilized egg in the fallopian tubes.

Some women with an ectopic pregnancy experience early signs of pregnancy such as a missed period, breast tenderness and nausea. The results of a pregnancy test will be positive.

Often the first warning signs of an ectopic pregnancy are pelvic pain and light vaginal bleeding. Other symptoms may include headaches and abdominal pain at mid-cycle.

With an ectopic pregnancy, the fertilized egg cannot survive. If it continues to grow in the fallopian tube, it can lead to the rupture of the tube. Heavy bleeding inside the abdomen is likely with symptoms of lightheadedness, fainting, severe abdominal pain and shock.

This is a life-threatening condition that may require emergency surgery or an injection of methotrexate to stop cell growth. This can lead to residual blockage of the fallopian tubes and subsequent infertility.

Chinese medicine can help prevent an ectopic pregnancy from occurring. It can also help in the recovery of full reproductive health after the completion of a Western medical procedure to address an ectopic pregnancy. Acupuncture administered in conjunction with herbal medicine enhances tubal patency after an ectopic pregnancy by reducing the size of obstructions in the fallopian tubes.

Possible Treatment Points
Sp 4 & PC 6 - Opens Chong Mai to reduce Blood Stasis.
Liv 3 - Moves Liver Qi. Invigorates Blood. Drains Damp Heat from the Lower Burner.
Ren 3, Ren 4 & Ren 6 - Use together help relieve menstrual pain.
Ren 3 - Regulates the Uterus & menstruation, clears Heat, relieves menstrual pain, & benefits the circulation of Qi & Blood. It also strengthens the Kidneys & helps with the retention of the placenta.
Ren 4 tonifies Original Qi & Kidneys. Calms the Spirit. Regulates the Uterus & promotes fertility. Treats lower abdominal pain.
Ren 6 tonifies Original Qi. Generates Qi & Yang. Expels Dampness. Invigorates Blood. Treats vaginal discharge & abdominal pain.
Sp 6 - Nourishes, harmonizes & invigorates Blood. Treats heavy & prolonged uterine bleeding during periods, Blood Stasis, Kidney Deficiency, Phlegm Dampness & Liver Qi Stagnation.
Sp 8 - Tonifies & invigorates Blood. Transforms Dampness. Regulates the Uterus.
St 25 - (Large Intestine Mu Point) - Clears Dampness & damp Heat & eliminates stasis in the Lower Abdomen. Regulates Blood & Qi.
St 29 - Warms the Lower Jiao. Invigorates Blood & regulates menstruation.
Zi Gong – Nourishes Essence & fertility. Brings Qi & Blood to the Uterus. Treats lower abdominal pain due to obstruction of Qi & Blood.

Acupuncture for Male Infertility

1. Erectile Dysfunction
2. Premature Ejaculation
3. Low Sperm Count
4. Low Sperm Motility

In TCM, the Kidneys are the primary organ system responsible for reproduction, growth and aging. Kidney Qi Deficiency in males can lead to a low sperm count, lack of sexual desire, impotence and sexual dysfunction. Other imbalances affecting male fertility are Damp Heat in the Liver Channel or Lower Burner, Liver or Heart Blood Deficiency, and the Heart and Kidneys Not Communicating.

Common Treatment Points

Kid 3 (Yuan Source Point) – Nourishes Essence & tonifies Jing. Especially useful for relieving sexual tensions, semen leakage, fatigue & loss of libido.

Kid 10 (He Sea Point) – Impotence. Premature ejaculation. Testicular pain. Nourishes the Kidneys.

Kid 8 - Swelling & pain of the testicles. Regulates Conception & Penetrating Channels. Role in ***Shutting in the Essence*** (In females wrapping or holding the uterine Blood in place)

Du 1 – Sexual taxation. Seminal emission induced by fear and fright

Other Possible Points:

GB 41 & SJ 5 – Regulates the Girdle Vessel & drains Dampness

Sp 4 & PC 6 – Opens & regulates the Penetrating Vessel

Ren 4 – Tonifies Jing & Essence. Significant point for Erectile Dysfunction, impotence, uro-reproductive problems, & urinary incontinence.

Ren 6 (Sea of Qi) - Tonifies Kidneys & Yuan Qi. Important point for impotence, & male reproductive dysfunction. Strengthens the reproductive system, treating erectile dysfunction, seminal emission, night-time urination, hernia and uro-reproductive problems.

St 28 (Water Passage - Level with Ren 4) – Regulates body fluids. Retention of urine & feces. Almost exclusively used for excess patterns of obstruction

St 29 (Level with Ren 3. Treat with Moxa or FIL) - Warms the Lower Jiao. Treats impotence, testicular & penile pain, pain in scrotum & seminal emissions.
St 36 – Transforms Dampness. Tonifies Original Qi. Strengthens the whole body & improves functioning of the sexual reproductive systems
Du 4 – Warms Gate of Vitality
BL 23 – Tonifies Jing & Yuan Qi. Treats impotency, premature ejaculation & sexual reproductive problems.
BL 27 & BL 34 - Essential points for male dysfunction treatment. Useful for treating impotency & sexual reproductive problems.
Kid 1 - Erectile dysfunction.

1. Erectile Dysfunction
Factors Affecting Erection
Du Mai, Kidney Yang, Fire of the Ming Men, Heart Blood, Chong Mai or Sea of Blood, Liver channel which wraps around pens, pathogenic factors such as Dampness, Blood Stasis, Stasis of Jing.

1.1 Kidney Yang Deficiency

Signs & Symptoms

- Impotence
- Lower backache
- Dizziness
- Tinnitus
- Frequent-pale urination
- Frequent night-time urination
- Feeling cold
- Cold lower back and knees
Tongue: Pale
Pulse: Deep, Weak.

Possible Acupuncture Points
SI 3 on the left & **BL 62** on the right - Opens the Du Mai
BL 23 (Kidney Shu) - Firms Kidney Qi. Benefits Essence
Du 20 - Tonifies Yang. Raises sinking Qi. Uplifting
Ren 6 (Sea of Qi) – Tonifies Yang & Original Qi
Ren 4 - Tonifies Jing, Essence & Yang Qi

Ren 3 - Dispels stagnation & drains Damp Heat
Kid 3.- Tonifies Jing & Kidney Yang. Treats impotence, seminal emissions, premature ejaculation.

1.2 Kidney Yin Deficiency

Signs & Symptoms

- Impotence
- Lower backache
- Dizziness
- Tinnitus
- Scanty-dark urine
- Night-sweating
- Insomnia
Tongue: Without coating
Pulse: Floating, Empty

Possible Acupuncture Points
SI 3 on the left **& BL 62** on the right – Opens Du Mai
LU 7 & Kid 6   - Opens Ren Mai
BL 23 (Kidney Shu) - Firms Kidney Qi. Benefits Essence
Du 20 - Tonifies Yang. Raises sinking Qi. Uplifting
Ren 6 (Sea of Qi) - Tonifies Yang & Original Qi
Ren 4 - Tonifies Jing, Essence & Yang Qi
Ren 3 - Dispels stagnation & drains Damp Heat
Kid 3 - Tonifies Jing & Kidney Yang. Treats impotence, seminal emissions & premature ejaculation.

1.3 Damp Heat in the Lower Burner

Signs & Symptoms

- Impotence
- Difficult, painful urination
- Turbid urine
- Itching of genitals
- Urethral discharge
Tongue: Sticky-yellow coating with red spots on root
Pulse: Slippery

Possible Acupuncture Points
SP 4 on the left **& PC 6** on the right - Opens Chong Mai
Liv 5 - Drains damp Heat from the Lower Burner. Moves Qi & Opens obstructions.
SP 9 – Drains damp Heat from the Lower Burner. Tonifies the Spleen
SP 6 – Transforms Dampness. Tonifies the Spleen. Invigorates Blood.
Ren 2 – Expels Wind Damp & warms the Kidneys
Ren 3 (Bladder Mu Pt) – Drains damp Heat. Tonifies the Kidneys
Liv 1 – Drains damp heat & moves Liver Qi
Liv 3 – Drains damp Heat from the Lower Burner. Moves Liver Qi.

1.4 Damp Heat in the Liver Channel

Signs & Symptoms:
- Impotence
- Difficult, painful urination
- Rash on external genitalia
- Irritability
Tongue: Red sides with sticky-yellow coating & red spots on the root
Pulse: Wiry

Possible Acupuncture Points
SP 4 on the left **& PC 6** on the right - Opens Chong Mai
Liv 5 - Drains Damp Heat from the Lower Burner. Moves Qi & Opens obstructions.
SP 9 - Drains Damp Heat from the Lower Burner. Tonifies the Spleen
SP 6 - Transforms Dampness. Tonifies the Spleen. Invigorates Blood.
Ren 2 - Expels Wind Damp & warms the Kidneys
Ren 3 (Bladder Mu Point) - Drains damp Heat. Tonifies the Kidneys.
Liv 1 - Drains damp Heat & moves Liver Qi
Liv 3 - Drains damp Heat from the Lower Burner. Moves Liver Qi.

1.5 Liver Blood Deficiency

Signs & Symptoms
- Impotence
- Dizziness
- Blurred vision
- Depression

- Insomnia
Tongue: Pale
Pulse: Choppy

Possible Acupuncture Points
LU 7 on the left & **Kid 6** on the right - Opens Ren Mai. Nourishes Kidney Yin.
BL 23 (Kidney Shu) - Tonifies Jing & Yuan Qi. Builds Blood.
Ren 4 - Tonifies Jing & Essence
Liv 8 - Nourishes & invigorates Blood. Tonifies the Liver & Kidneys.
Ren 3 (Bladder Mu Point) - Drains Damp Heat. Tonifies the Kidneys.
ST 36 - Builds Blood. Tonifies Original Qi.
SP 6 - Builds & invigorates Blood

1.6 Heart & Gall Bladder Qi Deficiency

Signs & Symptoms:
- Impotence
- Premature ejaculation
- Depression
- Timidity
- Sighing
- Insomnia
- Palpitations
- Easily startled
Tongue: Pale
Pulse: Weak

Possible Acupuncture Points
SI 3 on the left **& BL 62** on the right – Opens Du Mai (GV)
HE 7 - Tonifies the Heart & Heart Blood
GB 40 - Invigorates flow of Qi in the channel. Spreads Liver Qi & clears Gallbladder Heat.
Ren 4 - Tonifies Kidneys, Jing & Essence. Builds Blood.
Du 20 - Raises sinking Qi at lower end of the Du Mai
ST 36 - Builds Blood. Tonifies Original Qi.
SP 6 - Harmonizes the Liver & tonifies the Kidneys. Builds & invigorates Blood.

1.7 Heart Blood Deficiency

Signs & Symptoms
- Impotence
- Palpitations
- Dizziness
- Depression
- Insomnia

Tongue: Pale
Pulse: Choppy

Possible Acupuncture Points
SI 3 on the left & **BL 62** on the right – Opens Du Mai (GV)
HE 7 - Tonifies the Heart & Heart Blood
HE 5 - Calms the Spirit. Clears false Heat. Regulates Heart Fire & Qi.
Du 24 - Calms the Spirit. Lowers Liver Yang
Ren 15 - Calms the Spirit. Regulates Heart Qi.
Ren 4 - Tonifies Jing & Essence. Builds Blood.
Ren 3 - (Bladder Mu Point) - Tonifies the Kidneys. Clears Heat
BL 15 (Heart Shu Point) - Tonifies the Heart. Clears the Mind & Heart Fire
SP 6 - Harmonizes the Liver & tonifies the Kidneys. Builds & invigorates Blood.

1.8 Stasis of Jing & Phlegm

General Symptoms
- Impotence
- Pain in the testis and perineum
- Hypogastric pain
- Premature graying of hair
- Abnormal sperm (motility, shape, etc.)
- Oppression of the chest
- Urethral discharge
- Sweaty genitals

Male genital manifestations of Stasis of Jing

Although it may seem odd to talk of "Stasis" of Jing, it occurs in men and it is basically men's equivalent of Stasis of Blood in the Uterus.

The clinical manifestations of stasis of Jing are:
- Stabbing pain in the lumbar region
- Pain in the perineum
- Hypogastric pain
- Pain in the testis and/or penis
- Erectile dysfunction
- Premature ejaculation
- Priapism (persistent and painful erection of the penis.)
- Prostatic hypertrophy (enlarged prostate gland surrounding urethra)
- Premature graying of hair
- Itching or pain in the pubic region
- Peyronie's Disease (connective tissue disorder involving the growth of fibrous plaques in the soft tissue of the penis affecting about to 5% of men)
- Abnormal sperm

Tongue: Purple
Pulse: Firm, Slippery

Possible Acupuncture Points
SP 4 on the left & **P 6** on the right - Opens Chong Mai
Ren 3 - (Bladder Mu Point) – Drains Damp Heat. Tonifies the Kidneys
Ren 4 - Tonifies Jing, Essence & Yin & Yang Qi
Liv 5 - Drains Damp Heat from the Lower Burner. Moves Qi & opens obstructions.
SP 10 – Builds & cools Blood. Improves circulation of fluids.
BL 34 – Swelling & pain of the testicles
ST 40 – Expels Phlegm
SP 9 – Opens waterways in the Lower Burner. Transforms Dampness.

2. Premature Ejaculation

The Kidneys and Heart mutually support each other. The Kidneys belong to Water and the Heart to Fire. The Kidney Yin nourishes and moistens the Heart Yin, restraining Heart Fire. The Heart Yang descends to warm the Kidneys. When the Kidneys and Heart do not communicate the Spirit becomes agitated.

2.1 Heart & Kidneys Not Communicating
(Heart & Kidney Yin Deficiency)

Signs & Symptoms
- Premature ejaculation
- Five-Palm Heat
- Dizziness
- Tinnitus
- Night-sweating
- Palpitations
- Lower backache
- Depression.

Tongue: Red with no coating.
Pulse: Floating. Empty

Possible Acupuncture Points
SI 3 on the left **& BL 62** on the right - Opens Du Mai
HE 7 - Calms & Regulates the Spirit. Tonifies Heart Blood & Yin
Kid 7 - Strengthens Kidney function of dominating body fluids. Controls sweating.
Ren 15 - Calms the Spirit. Regulates Heart Qi. Clears Heat
Du 20 - Calms the Spirit. Raises sinking Qi
BL 23 - Nourishes the Essence. Builds Blood.
BL 32 - Tonifies Kidneys. Invigorates the Blood
Ren 4 - Tonifies Original Qi & Yin. Builds Blood
Kid 1 – Treats disharmony of Heart & Kidneys. Tonifies Yin.

2.2 Heart & Kidneys Not Communicating
(Heart & Kidney Qi Deficiency)

Signs & Symptoms:
- Premature ejaculation
- Dizziness
- Tinnitus
- Palpitations
- Lower backache
- Depression
- Pale face

Tongue: Pale, often enlarged, scalloped
Pulse: Weak or irregular. Often deep at Kidneys.

Possible Acupuncture Points
SI 3 on the left & **BL 62** on the right - Opens Du Mai
HE 7 - Calms & regulates the Spirit. Tonifies Heart Blood & Yin.
Kid 7 - Tonifies the Kidneys. Controls sweating.
Ren 15 - Calms the Spirit. Regulates Heart Qi. Benefits Yuan Qi.
Du 20 - Calms the Spirit. Raises sinking Qi. Tonifies Yang Qi
BL 23 - Nourishes the Essence, Yuan & Yang Qi.
BL 32 - Tonifies Kidneys. Invigorates the Blood.
Ren 4 - Tonifies Original Qi & Yin. Builds Blood
Kid 1 - Treats disharmony of Heart & Kidneys.

3. Low Sperm Count

3.1 Kidney Yang Deficiency

Signs & Symptoms
- Low sperm count
- Dizziness
- Tinnitus
- Lower backache
- Cold back and knees
- Frequent, pale urination
Tongue: Pale
Pulse: Weak, Deep

Possible Acupuncture Points
SI 3 on the left & **BL 62** on the right - Opens Du Mai
BL 23 (Kidney Shu) - Nourishes the Essence, Yuan & Yang/Yin Qi.
Ren 4 - Tonifies Jing, Essence & Yang/Yin Qi. Builds Blood.
Kid 13 - Tonifies Kidneys, Jing & Essence. Harmonizes Ren & Chong Channels
Kid 12 - Tonifies Kidneys & Yuan Qi. Harmonizes Ren & Chong Channels
BL 32 - Tonifies the Kidneys. Invigorates Blood
Kid 3 - Tonify Kidneys & Kidney Yang
Kid 7 - Tonify Kidney Yang

3.2 Kidney Yin Deficiency

Signs & Symptoms
- Low sperm count
- Dizziness
- Tinnitus
- Feeling of heat in the evening
- Night sweats
- Backache

Tongue: Without coating
Pulse: Floating, Empty

Possible Acupuncture Points
LU 7 on the left **& Kid 6** on the right – Opens Ren Mai. Nourishes Kidney Yin.
Ren 4 - Tonifies Jing, Essence & Yang/Yin Qi. Builds Blood.
Ren 7 - Tonifies The Kidneys & Yin Qi. Benefits the genital region – pain, retraction, damp itching or sweating of the testicles
Kid 13 - Tonifies Kidneys, Jing & Essence. Harmonizes Ren & Chong Channels.
Kid 12 - Tonifies Kidneys & Yuan Qi. Harmonizes Ren & Chong Channels
BL 23 (Kid Shu Point) - Nourishes the Essence, Yuan & Yang/Yin Qi.
Kid 3 - Tonify Kidneys. Nourishes Kidney Yin.
SP 6 - Nourish Yin

3.3 Liver Qi Stagnation with Kidney Deficiency

Signs & Symptoms
- Low sperm count
- Lower backache
- Dizziness
- Tinnitus
- Night-sweating
- Irritability
- Abdominal distension

Tongue: Without coating
Pulse: Weak & slightly Wiry on the left.

Possible Acupuncture Points
LU 7 on the left & **Kid 6** on the right – Opens Ren Mai
Ren 4 - Tonifies Jing, Essence & Yang/Yin Qi. Builds Blood.
Kid 13 - Tonifies Kidneys, Jing & Essence. Harmonizes Ren & Chong Channels.
Kid 12 - Tonifies Kidneys & Yuan Qi. Harmonizes Ren & Chong
BL 23 (Kidney Shu Point) - Nourishes the Essence, Yuan & Yang/Yin Qi.
Liv 3 - Moves Liver Qi & invigorates the Blood

3.4 Damp Heat in the Genital System

Signs & Symptoms
- Low sperm count
- Low motility
- Difficult urination
- Turbid urine
- Dark urine
- Painful urination
Tongue: Sticky, yellow coating with red spots at the root.
Pulse: Slippery

Possible Acupuncture Points
LU 7 on the left & **Kid 6** on the right - Opens Ren Mai
Ren 9 - Expels Dampness. Regulates water passages. Tonifies the Spleen.
ST 28 - Regulates water passages. Promotes urination. Tonifies the Kidneys.
Kid 12 - Tonifies Kidneys & Yuan Qi. Harmonizes Ren & Chong.
Ren 3 (Bladder Mu Point) - Drains Damp Heat. Promotes urination. Tonifies the Kidneys.
Ren 5 (San Jiao Mu Point) - Regulates water passages. Promotes urination. Tonifies Yang.
BL 22 (San Jiao Shu Point) - Drains Damp Heat from the Lower Burner. Regulates water passages. Tonifies the Spleen.
SP 9 - Drains Damp Heat from the Lower Burner. Tonifies the Spleen.
Liv 3 - Moves Liver Qi & Drains Damp Heat form the Lower Burner

3.5 Qi Stagnation & Blood Stasis

Signs & Symptoms
- Low sperm count
- Poor motility
- Distension and discomfort of testis
- Pain in the perineum
- Hypogastric pain
- Prostatic hypertrophy (enlarged prostate gland that surrounds the urethra)

Tongue: Purple
Pulse: Irregular, Knotted, Slow

Possible Acupuncture Points
SP 4 on the left & **PC 6** on the right – Opens Chong Mai
Liv 3 - Moves Liver Qi & invigorates the Blood. Drains Damp Heat from the Lower Burner.
SP 10 – Cools, builds & moves Blood. Removes stasis.
BL 17 (Diaphragm Shu Point) – Cools & builds Blood
Kid 14 – Regulates Qi, Blood & the Triple Burner
ST 30 – Builds & invigorates Blood. Invigorates the flow of Yuan Qi to the genitals.

4. Low Sperm Motility

4.1 Kidney Yang Deficiency

Signs & Symptoms
- Low sperm motility
- Impotence or sterility
- Pale, bright face. May also be darkish.
- Dizziness
- Backache
- Pale, frequent urination
- Premature ejaculation

Tongue: Pale, enlarged, scalloped. Moist with white thin fur.
Pulse: Frail and/or slow

Possible Acupuncture Points

SI 3 on the left **& BL 62** on the right – Opens Du Mai
BL 23 (Kidney Shu Point) - Nourishes the Essence, Yuan & Yang/Yin Qi
Ren 4 - Tonifies Jing, Essence & Yang/Yin Qi. Builds Blood.
Kid 13 - Tonifies Kidneys, Jing & Essence. Harmonizes Ren & Chong Channels. Strengthens the Chong Mai.
Kid 12 - Tonifies Kidneys & Yuan Qi. Harmonizes Ren & Chong Mai
BL 32 - Tonifies the Kidneys. Invigorates Blood
Kid 3 - Tonify Kidneys & Kidney Yang
Kid 7 - Tonify Kidney Yang

4.2 Kidney Yin Deficiency with Empty Heat

Signs & Symptoms
- Low sperm motility
- Backache
- Dizziness
- Tinnitus
- Night-sweating
- Five-Palm Heat
- Malar flush
- Nocturnal emissions with dreams
Tongue: Red without coating
Pulse: Floating, Empty & Rapid

Possible Acupuncture Points
LU 7 on the left & **Kid 6** on the right – Opens Ren Mai
Ren 4 - Tonifies Jing, Essence & Yang/Yin Qi. Builds Blood.
Kid 12 - Tonifies Kidneys & Yuan Qi. Harmonizes Ren & Chong Channels
HE 6 - Clears False Heat. Nourishes Yin.
Kid 3 - Tonify Kidneys. Nourishes Kidney Yin.
Ren 7 -Tonifies the Kidneys & Yin Qi. Benefits the genital region – pain, retraction, damp itching or sweating of the testicles
SP 6 - Nourish Yin. Builds Blood. Tonifies the Kidneys.

The Stress Challenge

Chronic emotional, physical and environmental stress creates obstacles to conception. Worry, overwork, poor diet, and an unhealthy lifestyle all contribute to increasing levels of stress.

Infertility often creates one of the most distressing life crises for couples and can generate deep feelings of loss. Patients find themselves feeling anxious, depressed, out of control, or socially isolated.

If infertility patients experience any of the following symptoms over a prolonged period, they could benefit from spending time with a mental health professional.

- Difficulty falling asleep or staying asleep, early morning awakening, sleeping more than usual
- Persistent feelings of pessimism, guilt, worthlessness, bitterness or anger
- Loss of interest in normal activities
- Depression that doesn't seem to go away
- Increased use of drugs or alcohol
- Thoughts about death or suicide
- Strained interpersonal relationships with partner, family, friends, or colleagues
- Difficulty thinking about anything other than infertility
- High levels of anxiety

There are certain points during infertility treatment when talking to a mental health professional can help patients deal with strained interpersonal relationships. Sharing one's fears and expectations can also help the couple choose the right medical treatment or explore other family building options.

When people are under stress, the hormone cortisol is released in the brain altering the brain's neurochemical balance. This changes hormone levels and disrupts the Hypothalamus-Pituitary-Ovarian Axis, which is key to the reproductive cycle.

Stress can prevent a woman from ovulating entirely. Stress can also create spasms in both the fallopian tubes and the Uterus, which can interfere with movement and implantation of a fertilized egg.

Stress can also affect men's ability to conceive altering sperm counts and motility and can also cause impotence.

Stress, anxiety, depression and other strong emotions interrupt the flow of energy. Over the long-term chronic stress can lead to disease and disorder.

Acupuncture helps patients relax, eliminating tension and obstacles to the smooth flow of Qi and Blood. This fosters a rebalancing of the energy, allowing the patient to enjoy an optimal state of health.

In addition, by improving circulation of Qi and Blood throughout the body, acupuncture helps oxygenate the tissues and eliminate cortisol and other waste chemicals. It releases natural pain-killing chemicals in the brain, called endorphins. The calming nature of acupuncture also decreases the Heart rate, lowers blood pressure and relaxes the muscles.

Integrating Acupuncture and Chinese herbal medicine with a healthy diet and lifestyle creates balance, which in turn enhances fertility.

Dietary Recommendations

The nutrients that circulate throughout the body have a profound effect on the function of the reproductive organs. One of the most important things a person can do to become pregnant is to choose fertile foods and a healthy lifestyle.

Western nutrition categorizes foods according to their vitamin and mineral content. TCM factors in the energetic qualities of foods and their impact on the body's overall energetic balance.

Excessive consumption of cold foods may create Cold in the Uterus while excessive consumption of hot foods may cause Blood Heat and therefore heavy periods

A diet lacking in nourishment may lead to Qi and Blood Deficiency which can result in scanty periods, absence of periods, or infertility.

Eat primarily organic with less animal protein and more vegetable protein. Increase consumption of:

- Dark leafy green vegetables and fruits
- Legumes and their sprouts
- Fresh Nuts and Seeds
- Seaweed

Also do not overeat, prepare you own food and enjoy eating.

To Avoid

For optimum fertility, limit or avoid exposure to chemicals, heavy metals, antibiotics, hormones and the following items:

- Animal products with hormones and antibiotics
- Junk food and candy
- Refined or processed oils
- Large fish (Tuna and Halibut)
- Coffee
- Cold foods such as raw fruits and vegetable and cold drinks or food

from the fridge which lead to invasion of Cold in the Uterus. This happens more commonly in puberty, during menstruation and after birthing.
- Hot foods such as meats, spices, as well as alcohol and smoking, which can lead to stagnation of Liver Qi and Blood Heat.
- Greasy foods such as dairy products, peanuts, fatty meats, fried foods, sweets and sugar which can cause accumulation of Dampness or Phlegm that often settles in the Lower Burner causing painful periods, excessive vaginal discharge or cysts.
- Processed foods or an unbalanced diet which can lead to Deficiency of Qi and Blood as well as Dampness.
- Sour foods such as yoghurt, vinegar, pickles, oranges and orange juice, grapefruit and grapefruit juice, gooseberries, black currants and red currants. Because of the astringent nature of these foods, they may stop bleeding if eaten during the menses.
- Strongly scented bath oils, incense, candles, lotions and perfumes

Diet per Menstrual Cycle

Menstruation

Because of the loss of Blood, menstruation is a good time to focus on Blood nourishing foods that are rich in iron such as black beans, fish, leafy green vegetables and seeds. Most of these foods are rich in iron, protein or both, which is especially important for women with endometriosis or heavy bleeding.

Other foods that nourish Blood are egg yolks, liver, beef, chicken, carrots, spinach, wood-ear mushrooms, peanuts and Chinese red dates.

Fish, seeds and leafy greens have anti-inflammatory properties, which can help mitigate cramps by encouraging healthy Blood flow.

Eat plenty of bell peppers, tomatoes, broccoli, kiwi, citrus and other food sources that are high in vitamin C. Vitamin C helps the body absorb iron from beans, whole grains and fortified cereals.

Avoid cold foods if periods are clotted and painful as well as alcohol, caffeine and spicy foods, which can make bleeding heavier.

Follicular Phase

During the follicular phase, the body is working hard to develop a dominant follicle and estrogen levels are on the rise. Unfortunately, women who are struggling with fibroids and endometriosis often have too much estrogen (a condition called estrogen dominance).

Veggies like broccoli, kale, cabbage and cauliflower contain a phytonutrient which helps women metabolize estrogen and help rid the body of environmental estrogen absorbed from the pesticides and hormones found in meat and dairy products.

Focus on foods that support follicle development like green vegetables, legumes, eggs, fish, olive oil, avocado, nuts and seeds. These foods are loaded with vitamin E, which is found in the fluid of the follicle that houses the eggs.

Avoid alcohol as it affects hormonal balance. Alcohol is also dehydrating. The loss of water in the body may thicken the cervical mucus.

Ovulation Phase

Close to ovulation, the body needs plenty of B vitamins and other nutrients to support the release of the egg and promote implantation. Vitamin C is found in high quantities in the follicle after the egg is released and may play a role in progesterone production. Zinc can help with cell division and progesterone production.

Essential fatty acids (EFAs) are also crucial during this phase. Fish oil provides the best source of omega-3s. EFAs promote Blood flow to the Uterus, support the opening of the follicle facilitating the release of the egg, and open the tiny Blood vessels in the groin area. Fish oil thins out Blood, increases circulation and boosts testosterone levels.

Focus on leafy greens, whole grains, eggs, legumes, fish and water which plays a key role in transporting hormones and in developing follicles. It also helps thin out cervical mucus, which may make it a little easier for the sperm to reach the egg.

Avoid acidic foods like coffee, alcohol, meat and processed foods, which may make the cervical mucus hostile to sperm. Alkaline foods are a smarter choice, particularly green vegetables, sprouts and wheatgrass.

Luteal Phase

The luteal phase is all about creating higher temperatures to help maintain pregnancy. Promote growth and expansion by focusing on warming foods like soups and stews. Avoid cold or raw foods, especially ice cream and frozen yogurt as cold constricts.

During the Luteal Phase it is important to consume nutrients that encourage cell growth. Beta-carotene, which is commonly found in leafy greens as well as in yellow and orange foods (e.g., carrots, cantaloupe and sweet potatoes), helps keep hormones in check and prevents early miscarriage.

In fact, the corpus luteum, which helps produce the progesterone necessary to sustain a pregnancy, is loaded with beta-carotene.

Pineapple gets a lot of attention during this phase. It contains bromelain, which has been shown to mildly support implantation through its anti-inflammatory properties.

Herbs and Pregnancy

Herbal Medicine stimulates the production of hormones naturally by the body. Specialised herbal formulas can also alter the rate of hormone metabolism and change the response of hormone receptors, helping the body produce the proper levels of hormones.

It is important to consult a trained and experienced herbalist if you want to take herbs to enhance fertility or enjoy a healthy pregnancy. Your medical doctor should be consulted to ensure proper coordination with any medical treatments being offered.

Patients should never self-diagnose or self-dose with herbal medicine as some herbal products may contain agents that are contraindicated in pregnancy that could lead to miscarriage, premature birth, uterine contractions, or injury to the fetus.

Herbal Formulas

Herbal medicine for fertility offers a variety of treatment approaches and, combined with acupuncture, substantially increase chances of a successful pregnancy. The general approach is to boost Blood and Kidney Qi, and address any specific problems affecting fertility.

Herbal formulas are available to support the four phases of the menstrual cycle. During the Menstrual Phase the herbal formula is especially effective in treating Blood Stasis. It opens the collaterals to eliminate Blood Stasis and facilitates the complete discharge of the endometrial lining.

During the Follicular Phase the herbal formula regulates the length of the phase, increases cervical mucus, improves the quantity and quality of menstrual Blood, regulates basal body temperature, and improves the development of follicles and the endometrial lining.

During the Ovulation Phase the herbal formula invigorates Blood and remove Blood Stasis, while promoting a healthy Yin foundation, and the ability of Yang to mobilize at ovulation. Herbs are more powerful in strengthening Yin than acupuncture.

During the Luteal Phase the herbal formula tonifies and invigorates the Yang and Spleen Qi. Additional herbs are often added to support Yin and Blood, to move Liver Qi Stagnation, and to calm the Spirit.

Adding the appropriate herbal formulas to treatment significantly increases the chances of becoming pregnant for women and of improving the quality of sperm for men. Achieving a successful pregnancy may be quick, within one or two months, or prolonged over six to eight months. The best sign of progress is the gradual improvement of menstrual issues. This particularly applies to irregular periods or amenorrhea.

Western medicine does not have a lot of treatment options to offer for problems with sperm motility or sperm morphology. Chinese herbs and acupuncture can effectively enhance sperm quality in general and are especially useful when tests show issues with suboptimal sperm. It takes three months for new sperm to grow and develop naturally. Therefore, the herbal formula must be taken for the full three months before retesting the sperm.

Additional herbal formulas are often used to address specific women's issues such as a Cold Uterus, Stagnation of Dampness and Phlegm, PMS, or overgrowth of reproductive tissues.

In cases of menstrual cramping, adding a formula during or before cramping may be necessary starting a day or so before cramping begins, and continuing until cramping and clot expulsion is finished.

After the age of 39, the viability of the woman's eggs diminishes. This is a common reason for first-trimester miscarriage in older women. Chinese herbs cannot strengthen the life-force or integrity of the egg. Also herbal formulas should not be taken when the patient is undergoing hormonal therapy except for progesterone augmentation.

Frequent miscarriages often accompany infertility, and in modern medicine this is correlated with low levels of progesterone. Herbal formulas that build Blood and Kidney Qi also boost progesterone levels. It is helpful to continue with Blood tonics during the first trimester, to boost progesterone and help prevent miscarriage.

A complete health history will help identify the appropriate herbal formula or formulas that best fits the patient's condition.

Individual Herbal Supplements

The following herbal supplements are generally considered safe during pregnancy.

Red Raspberry Leaf – Rich in iron, this herb helps tone the Uterus, increase milk production, decrease nausea, and ease labor pains. It may also reduce complications during birth. Many health care providers only recommend using it after the first trimester.

Peppermint Leaf – Helpful in relieving nausea/morning sickness and flatulence.

Ginger root – Helps relieve nausea and vomiting.

Slippery Elm Bark – Used to help relieve nausea, heartburn, and vaginal irritations when the inner bark is used orally in similar amounts used in foods.

Oats and Oat Straw – Rich in calcium and magnesium. Helps relieve anxiety, restlessness, and irritated skin.

Dandelion – Rich in Vitamin A, calcium, and iron. Dandelion root and leaf can also help relieve mild edema and nourish the Liver

Chamomile (German) – High in calcium and magnesium. Helps with sleeplessness and inflammation of joints.

Nettles (Stinging Nettles) – High in vitamins A, C, K, calcium, potassium, and iron. Great all-around pregnancy tonic.

Vitamin B9 (Folic Acid) – Normalizes gestation during pregnancy. Helps prevent miscarriage and neural tube defects, the embryonic structure that develops into the baby's brain and spinal cord. Promotes Heart health and helps prevent anemia. Found in spinach, leafy greens, broccoli, mango, avocado, lentils, asparagus and oranges.

Qi Gong for Infertility

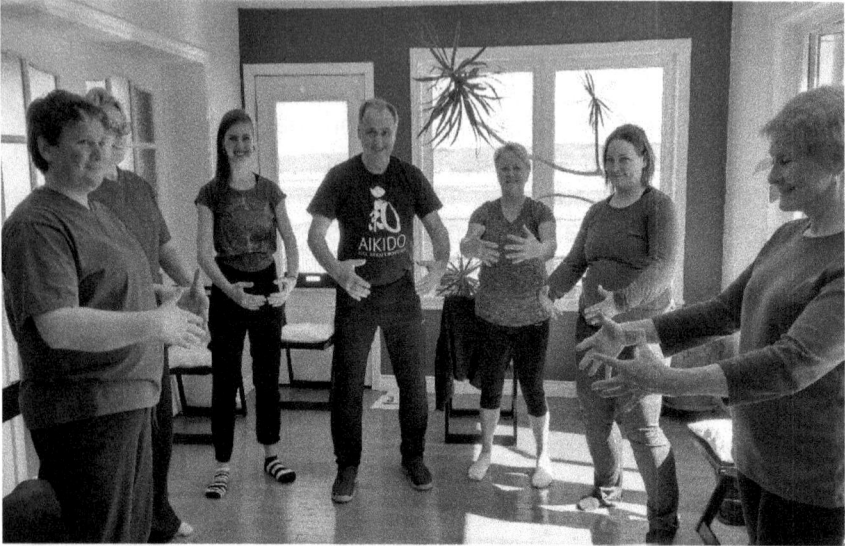

Qi Gong postural, breathing and visualisation exercises can facilitate fertility by helping to regulate the menstrual cycle and reduce obstructions in the female reproductive system. Qi Gong can also help both men and women increase their reproductive vitality by strengthening the Kidneys.

The following are a few basic exercises for your consideration. For more information please review my three books on Qi Gong entitled The Power of Qi for Health and Longevity, Qi Gong's Five Golden Keys, and Dance of the Dragon - Healing Oneself and Others.

Start all Qi Gong exercises with the following Relaxed Abdominal Breathing exercise.

Natural or Belly Breathing

First adopt a standing posture with the following indications:

Feet shoulder width apart, 70% of body weight on the heels, knees straight but soft, abdomen pressed gently against the lower back, chin in with Adam's apple raised slightly upward.

Arms hang down the sides of the body with the palms of the hands open and facing the sides of the body.

Anus is closed, and the tip of tongue gently placed on the upper palate behind the front teeth.

Align the three points: Crown of Head, Center of the Perineum, and the Midpoint of the line connecting the heels of the feet.

Drop the tailbone down. Open the Crown Point to the sky. Gently open the space between the shoulder blades.

Practice with soft eyes that are fully open, or half closed looking to the horizon.

Inhale through the nose, to the count of seven, expanding the lower part of the body, front, side and back. Exhale through the nose to the count of ten letting the chest drop down towards the hips.

The breath is gentle, silent, slow, deep and unbroken. Let the inhalation rise on its own from the space between exhalation and inhalation. Thirty breaths equal approximately five minutes.

Lighting the Fire in the Lower Dantian with Reverse Breathing

In Daoism the body is considered Yin and the eyes Yang. Look into the Lower Dantian or Lower Abdomen to start the fire and heat up Yin. It takes two to three months for a regular person to feel heat in the Lower Dantian.

Do not think too much. Stay in the center of the Lower Dantian for a few minutes but do not stare. Use the Mind's eye to plant the Qi seed and let it grow without effort.

The following exercise helps further energize the Lower Dantian. It involves reverse breathing and the gentle lifting of the anus and perineum. It is good for increasing sexual energy, for premature ejaculation, and for preventing prolapsed of the anus, Uterus and Stomach. It is also good for the excretory system and helps prevent hemorrhoids, colon cancer and localized infections.

Move 70% of the body's weight to the front third of the feet. Bring the palms to navel. Women right hand first, men left hand first. The hands can also rest in any position.

Inhale contracting the abdomen and gently lifting the anus. Exhale and relax, bringing the Mind to the Lower Dantian. Repeat 10 to 50 times.

On inhalation, visualize the energy moving in a circular fashion, like the turning of a wheel, from the navel to the Hui Yin (Pelvic Floor) to the Ming Men (Lower Back) and back to the navel where you exhale and relax.

Movement creates energy. If a space does not move it becomes stagnant and problems can result. Reverse breathing creates a smaller space in the abdomen. It moves the organs and creates more energy. It is a powerful exercise so proceed with caution starting with only 10 repetitions and increasing repetitions slowly over time to up to 50 per session.

This is a great exercise to strengthen men's Jing Qi and reproductive capability. Men can practice this at any time. Women who are trying to get pregnant should avoid doing this exercise during the Ovulation Phase and the first half of the Luteal Phase. Women should not do this exercise if pregnant.

Cleansing Breath in a Standing Posture

In a standing posture, arms hanging down the sides of the body, visualize breathing pure universal energy in through the Crown of the head, down the center core of the body, into the abdomen. Then breathe stagnant Qi out the legs and feet deep into the earth. Repeat 10 to 30 times.

If there is an obstruction in the reproductive organs, such as ovarian cysts or uterine fibroids, visualize breathing pure energy from the Universe via the pores of the skin into the Uterus and ovaries.

As you inhale, visualise that the congestion in the reproductive organs is breaking up. On exhalation send the debris from the breakup out of the body via the pores of the skin far into the Universe. Repeat 10 to 30 times.

Women should not practice this exercise during the menses if they are experiencing excessive bleeding. Men can practice this at any time.

Self-Massage to Clear Obstructions of the Female Reproductive Organs

Self-massage to the abdominal area between the navel and pubic bone can help break up adhesions in the reproductive organs. This self-massage technique can be done standing.

Divide the lower abdomen into three lines. One line connects the navel with the center of the pubic bone, the second is parallel to the first line about two thumb widths out and the third parallel to the center about three thumb widths out. Place the pads of the fingers on the first line just above the pubic bone.

Massage the area by applying firm pressure and turning the pads of the fingers in a counterclockwise direction 10 to 12 times before repeating the movement in a counterclockwise direction 10 to 12 times. Raise the fingers about a thumb-width and repeat. Then raise again another thumb width and repeat again.

Move back to the public bone about two thumb widths away from the center line and repeat the same sequence. Move the fingers down to the inguinal crease and massage three points on this line. Repeat on the opposite side.

Once the nine points have been massaged, with left hand over right, massage down each of the three lines the heel of the right hand applying moderate pressure 6 to 9 times each before letting the palms rest over the navel for a few minutes.

Energizing the Uterus

Move the hands away from the lower abdomen. Imagine the palms are holding a balloon or Qi ball. The hands are located about two fist widths away from the abdomen, at the same level as the Sea of Qi Point located just below the navel.

Breathe in pure Universal energy into the palms and exhale sending the energy from the palms into the reproductive organs. Imagine the Uterus being receptive, warm and vibrant. Practice for 10 to 20 minutes or until you feel warmth in the Uterus.

Closing Relaxation with Soong

Place the palms over the lower abdomen, thumbs overlapping slightly at the navel, men right hand over left, and women left hand over right. Bring the feet together so the heels touch.

Using the Mind, expand the body outward and inhale Universal Qi. Exhale with the sound SOONG vibrating the nose and whole body. Repeat 6 to 9 times.

Acupuncture for a Healthy Baby

Typically, most miscarriages occur within the first 3 months of pregnancy. Consequently, treatment of patients may often last through week twelve to help prevent miscarriage and longer if the patient is experiencing issues such as insomnia, nausea or abdominal pain. If ever a patient experiences signs of cramping, bleeding and low back pain during pregnancy she should seek medical help immediately.

The Beautiful Baby Point - Kid 9

There is an ancient Chinese acupuncture treatment that has been used for centuries to ensure a healthy, beautiful baby. Kidney 9 is gently stimulated with a golden needle. Gold is warm by nature and works well to strengthen the body and stimulate Qi.

The beautiful baby point is located above the medial malleolus (inner ankle bone), right below the calf muscle. Even though the acupuncture point is located on the lower leg, it is a powerful point that is connected to meridians throughout the body and is used to calm the Mind, and build or tonify Blood. It treats hypertension, fear, anxiety, nightmares, and mental disorders.

Suggested Auricular Points

Left Ear: Uterus & Endocrine Points
Right Ear: Shen Men & Brain acupuncture points.

Cautions:

1. When needling Ren 4, the needle should just reach the muscle level – don't insert it too deep.

2. Don't stimulate the points, just slightly reinforce their action. Over stimulation of the points might cause a miscarriage.

3. If you use heat lamp, don't put it too close to the lower abdominal and don't allow the patient to feel too hot in the lower abdominal area.

General Treatment Points
No Specific Issues
(Where applicable all points are bilateral)

Liv 3 - Calms the Spirit & Liver Fire. Stops bleeding. Moves Qi & Invigorates Blood

Kid 3 – Insomnia. Lower Back Pain. Nourishes Essence & Kidney Yin & Yang.

Kid 9 - Calms the Mind. Builds Blood. Creates a receptive environment in the Uterus for the baby.

Li 11 - Clears Damp Heat. Cools Blood. Benefits tendons & joints. Treats abdominal pain

HT 7 - Tonifies Heart Blood. Calms the Mind. Treats Insomnia.

Yin Tang (Mid-Eyebrow Point) - Calms the Spirit. Treats insomnia, anxiety & agitation.

PC 5 - Calms the Mind. Expels Dampness. Regulates the Uterus. Treats disorders of the Heart.

SP 1 - Tonifies the Spleen. Treats Uterine bleeding & abdominal disorders. Calms the Mind

Treatments for Common Issues
1st, 2nd, 3rd Trimesters

During pregnancy there is an abundance of Yin due to the absence of menses and the increase of fluids in the body. Pregnancy puts a strain on the Kidneys as their Qi and Essence go to feed the fetus. But the absence of menses provides additional Blood to feed the body and fetus.

Therefore, some heath conditions such as asthma and migraines often improve with pregnancy. Others experience a deterioration in their health during pregnancy depending on the pre-existing state of the Kidney Qi, and how well a woman looks after herself after pregnancy.

Contradictory symptoms of Hot and Cold often appear such as cold hands and feet with a feeling of Heat in the face.

These contradictory symptoms can be caused by:
- Yin Fire from Deficiency of Original Qi. Yin Deficiency may manifest

as Cold while the Yin Fire causes Hot Symptoms such as a feeling of Heat, low-grade fever, dry mouth and restless limbs.
- Empty Heat from Blood Deficiency which leads to cold hands and feet, and a feeling of Heat in the face with red cheekbones on a pale face.
- Rebellious Qi of the Chong Mai with a feeling of Heat in the face and cold in the feet.
- Severe Qi Stagnation causing a feeling of Heat in the face and cold hands and feet, as Qi obstructs the circulation of Qi in the channels.
- Kidney Yang deficiency and Heart Heat.

Previous patterns of weakness, overwork, negative emotions and poor lifestyle may lead to complications during the first trimester such as:

1. Threat of Miscarriage
2. Anxiety
3. Morning Sickness
4. Heartburn
5. Constipation
6. Hemorrhoids
7. Breech Baby

1. Threat of Miscarriage

Many pregnancy losses are caused by the same immunological factors and hormonal imbalances that are at the root of infertility. One of the most common reasons for a miscarriage is inadequate progesterone production, the same factor related to Luteal Phase Defect.

Slight vaginal bleeding which leads to more bleeding in the first trimester indicates a high likelihood of a miscarriage, especially if the bleeding progressively gets worse. Other indicators of a miscarriage according to TCM are "restless fetus", and "falling fetus". In general, there is a weakness of the Ren and Chong Meridians to gather Blood and nourish the fetus.

A miscarriage can be caused by:
- Foetal abnormalities which increase with age
- Weak sperm related to the age of the male
- Hormonal dysfunction

- Cervical, uterine or tubal abnormalities caused by fibroids, PSOS, endometriosis, etc.
- Congenital abnormalities of the Uterus

A deficiency in the Kidneys is most often behind these issues although, Blood Deficiency and Spleen Deficiency can also play a role. Problems may arise from overwork, strong emotions, trauma, and excessive sexual activity within the first three months of pregnancy.

Blood Stasis, poor circulation in the Uterus or scar tissue limit the appropriate sites of attachment of the embryo in the endometrial lining. This is best treated during the menses to ensure the thorough discharge and rebuilding of endometrial tissue. Proper treatment after the menses also helps the development of a thick lining.

It is important to track the BBT (Basil Body Temperature) for the first few weeks of pregnancy as it is indicative of appropriate Kidney Yang and progesterone levels required to maintain a healthy environment in the Uterus for the development of the foetus. For practitioners certified in Chinese Herbs, it is helpful to continue with Blood tonics during the first trimester, to boost progesterone levels and prevent miscarriage.

The treatment described below is for the threat of a miscarriage. Do not intervene if there is a miscarriage during first trimester as it is a natural occurrence of rejection and may be due to genetic damage. Normally, after 12 weeks the patient will be in the clear.

General Points for Recurrent Miscarriages
BL 26 (Back Shu point of Gate of Vitality) – All cases of Lower Back Pain, diarrhea
Kid 8 – Uterine bleeding & prolapse. Clears Heat & expels Dampness
Du 4 (moxibustion) – Warm the Gate of Vitality or Gate of Fire
ST 28 – Regulates water passages. Dispels stagnation in the Lower Jiao, Benefits the Uterus
Ren 6, Ren 7 – Tonifies Kidneys & Kidney Yin. Ren 6 tonifies upright Qi. Use only if there is a history of miscarriages. Counter indicated in second trimester.
Sp 1 with Moxa – Given as home care to help stop vaginal bleeding. Done every hour during the day for 15 minutes with a moxa stick.
Kid 2 (moxibustion) - Clears false Heat. Uterine prolapse

1.1 Kidney Deficiency (Vaginal bleeding issues)

Signs & Symptoms
- Scanty vaginal bleeding
- Lumbar soreness
- Dizziness
- Fatigue
- Frequent urination

Tongue: Pale (Kidney Yang), or Red with no Coating (Kidney Yin)
Pulse: Deep, Weak (Kidney Yang), or Floating, Empty (Kidney Yin)
Tx: Tonify Kidney, Strengthen the Governor, Conception and Chong Meridians, Calm the Fetus

Possible Acupuncture Points
BL 20 (Spleen Shu) – Tonifies Spleen
BL 23 (Kidney Shu) & **BL 17 (T7)** - Tonifies Kidneys & Blood
Kid 3 - Tonifies Kidneys
GV 20 - Raises energy, lifts fetus
SP 1 - Stops uterine bleeding
ST 36 - Tonifies Qi

1.2 Qi & Blood Deficiency (Vaginal bleeding issues)

Signs & Symptoms
- Vaginal bleeding (more at end of 1st trimester)
- Scanty pale and diluted Blood
- Weakness
- Fatigue
- Pale complexion
- Palpitations

Tongue: Pale
Pulse: Fine, weak, empty
Tx: Tonify Qi & Build Blood

Possible Acupuncture Points
ST 36 – Tonifies Qi
BL 20 (Spleen Shu) – Tonifies Spleen
BL 23 (Kidney Shu) – Tonifies Kidneys
BL 17 (Sea of Blood) **& BL 19** (Gallbladder Shu) -"Four flowers", Builds Blood

154

Liv 8 - Tonifies Blood
SP 1 - Stops uterine bleeding

1.3 Blood Heat (Vaginal bleeding issues)

Signs and Symptoms
- Scanty vaginal bleeding
- Bright red Blood
- Sensations of heat
- Abdominal pain
- Thirst
- Constipation
- Anxiety
- Insomnia
- Dark urine
Tongue: Red with Yellow Coating
Pulse: Rapid, Full
Tx: Clear Heat, Cool Blood, Calm the Fetus

Possible Acupuncture Points
Liv 2 - Clears Heat
LI 11 & SP 10 - Clears Heat. Cools Blood.
Kid 2 - Clears Heat
Liv 3 - Regulates Liver
SP 1 - Stops uterine bleeding

2. Anxiety

Everyone suffers from anxiety from time to time. But when anxiety takes over with physical symptoms such as nausea, fatigue, heart palpitations and insomnia, it can become a major health issue and severely impact one's quality of life.

Anxiety is often driven by feelings of worry, fear, loss, or guilt. Often it is difficult to identify the exact origin of these negative emotions.

Prescription drugs can help ease anxiety but may also cause undesirable side effects by increasing the chemical toxicity of the body weakening the Liver which, in Chinese Medicine, plays an important role in harmonizing emotions.

Acupuncture, Herbal Medicine and Qi Gong relaxation exercises provide an effective and non-invasive alternative for the treatment of anxiety by promoting relaxation, strengthening the Liver's ability to harmonize the emotions, and deactivating the analytical brain, which is responsible for anxiety and worry.

Mild to moderate depression responds well to acupuncture, herbs and Qi Gong, which may be combined with conventional medication or used alone under proper supervision. In cases of severe depression, these modalities may be used to enhance conventional therapy.

2.1 Liver Fire

Signs & Symptoms
- Anxiety
- Mental restlessness
- Irritability
- Anger
- Dry mouth
- Thirst
- Red eyes
- Darker urine
- Constipation
- Dizziness
- Tinnitus
- Dream disturbed sleep

Tongue: Red with red sides. Dry Yellow coat
Pulse: Wiry, Rapid
Tx: Drain Liver Fire. Calm the Mind

Possible Acupuncture Points
Liv 2 - Drains Liver fire – lots of anger.
Liv 3 - Treats anxiety, palpitations & nervousness. Also useful in the treatment of insomnia & PMS.
Liv 3 & GB 41 - Soul healing points. Together they relieve irritability, & balance resentment, jealousy, anger, attitude problems & judgment.
Liv 8 - Tonifies the Liver & Clears Liver Fire & the Mind
BL 18 (Liver Shu Point) - Tonifies & sedates the Liver. Clears the Mind.
DU 18 - Calms the Mind. Sedates the Liver

HT 7 (Spirit Gate) – Promotes clarity of Mind. Relaxes the Mind & body. Regulates extremes of the Heart – ups & downs. Treats insomnia, chronic stress, nervousness, mania, annoyance, & depression. Relieves sadness & anxiety.
PC 7 – Calms the Mind. Clears Heat from the Heart. Treats mania, manic raving, ceaseless laughter, agitation, sadness, fright & fear, weeping with grief.
GB 13 – Prevents emotional extremes. Gathers Jing to the Brain. Works on Jing, Kidneys & Marrow. Root of the Shen. Makes Shen return to its root. Connects Shen & Jing, Heart & Kidneys.

2.2 Yin Deficiency (Empty Heat)

Signs & Symptoms
- Anxiety
- Mental restlessness
- Difficulty relaxing (particularly in the evening)
- Fidgety
- Palpitations
- Dry mouth
- Night sweats
Tongue: Red with no coat
Pulse: Rapid
Tx: Tonify Yin, Clear Empty Heat, Calm the Mind

Possible Acupuncture Points
Kid 2 - Clears Empty Heat
Kid 3 - Balances the Kidneys & tonifies Kidney Yin. Strengthens will power & the Brain. Treats fear. Stabilizes intimate relationships. Relieves feelings of abandonment & guilt. Treats issues emanating from incest.
Kid 6 - Tonifies Kidney Yin (fear)
HT 6 - Clears Empty Heat & night sweats
HT 7 (Spirit Gate) – Promotes clarity of Mind. Relaxes the Mind & body. Regulates extremes of the Heart – ups & downs. Treats insomnia, chronic stress, nervousness, mania, annoyance, & depression. Relieves sadness & anxiety.
BL 15 (Heart Shu) - Calms the Spirit. Anxiety. Night Sweats.

PC 7 – Calms the Mind. Clears Heat from the Heart. Treats mania, manic raving, ceaseless laughter, agitation, sadness, fright & fear, weeping with grief.

2.3 Phlegm Fire Harassing the Mind

Signs & Symptoms
- Strong agitation
- Phobias
- Irritability
- Chest oppression
- Nausea

Tongue: Red and Swollen, Sticky Coat
Pulse: Slippery, Rapid
Tx: Resolve Phlegm, Calm the Mind

Possible Acupuncture Points
ST 40 - Resolves Phlegm
SP 9 - Resolves Dampness
Liv 2 - Drains Fire. Promotes urination.
LI 11 - Clears Heat. Drains damp Heat
ST 8 - Clears the Head. Headaches due to Dampness.
GB 17 - Clears Heat & the Head. Lowers Liver Yang. Treats migraines, headaches, anxiety & dizziness due to phlegm-fluid.

Consider using auricular points **Shenmen** and **Zero Point.** If the patient is suffering from Qi Stagnation add **Ren 15** or **Ren 17**.

3. Morning Sickness

A change in the Uterus may reflect in the Stomach via the Chong Mai. The descending effect the Chong Mai has on the body may be disrupted leading to the counter flow of Stomach Qi and poor digestion. Emotionally, the Spleen is related to worry and overthinking, so an excess of these emotions may also disrupt the functioning of the Stomach and Spleen organ systems.

The pregnancy may be endangered if the vomiting becomes extreme or the Qi rises further along the Chong Mai affecting the Heart.

Ginger is an effective remedy for morning sickness. Even at doses as low as 1 gm per day, symptoms can be relieved. The ginger must be taken for a minimum of 48 hours to up to four days before it becomes effective.

General Symptoms
- Nausea
- Vomiting
- General lethargy
- Strong food cravings or aversions

3.1 Stomach and/or Spleen Qi Deficiency

Signs & Symptoms
- Slight morning sickness. If there is vomiting it may be small amounts & diluted.
- Poor appetite
- Fatigue
- Feeling of cold
- Depression is also possible

Tongue: Pale
Pulse: Weak
Tx: Harmonize & strengthen the Stomach & Spleen

Possible Acupuncture Points
SP 4 Right **& PC 6** Left - Regulates Chong Mai. Stops nausea & vomiting. (Only use if no history of miscarriage – otherwise use **PC 6** only)
ST 36 - Tonifies Stomach & Spleen Qi
Ren 10 - Retains food in the Stomach. Controls the cardiac sphincter of the Stomach.
Ren 12 -Tonifies Stomach & Spleen Qi. Improves down-bearing effect of Stomach Qi.
BL 20 (Spleen Shu) – Tonifies Stomach & Spleen Qi. Transforms Dampness.
BL 21 (Stomach Shu) – Tonifies Stomach Qi. Harmonizes the Middle Burner. Improves down-bearing effect of Stomach Qi. Expels Dampness.

3.2 Liver Qi Stagnation invading the Stomach

Signs & Symptoms
- Morning sickness with retching vomiting
- Sour taste in mouth
- Epigastric fullness
- Irritability

Tongue: Red Sides
Pulse: Wiry
Tx: Soothe the Liver. Relieve Stagnation. Descend Rebellious Qi.

Possible Acupuncture Points
PC 6 - Stop nausea/vomiting
Liv 14 (Front Liver Mu Point) – Regulates the Liver Qi, belching, heart burn, & rebellious Stomach Qi
ST 36 - Tonify Stomach & Spleen Qi
Ren 12 - Tonify Stomach & Spleen Qi
KD 21 - Regulate Chong Mai, morning sickness, digestive disorders, nausea, & vomiting.
ST 34 - Regulates Stomach. Stops vomiting.

3.3 Accumulation of Phlegm

Signs & Symptoms
- Profuse vomiting
- Signs of mucus & dampness
- Chest oppression
- Dizziness

Tongue: Swollen, Sticky Coat
Pulse: Slippery
Tx: Resolve Phlegm, Subdue Rebellious Qi

Possible Acupuncture Points
ST 40 - Resolves phlegm & dampness
SP 9 - Resolves dampness
PC 6 - Stops nausea
BL 20 (Spleen Shu Point) – Tonifies the Spleen. Expels Dampness.
Ren 12 - Tonifies Stomach & Spleen

3.4 Heart Qi Deficiency

Signs & Symptoms
- Morning sickness with palpitations
- Anxiety
Tongue: Pale
Pulse: Empty at Heart Position
Tx: Tonify Heart Qi. Calm the Mind. Regulate the Stomach

Possible Acupuncture Points
PC 6 - Stops nausea & vomiting
ST 36 - Tonifies Stomach & Spleen Qi
Ren 14 - Tonifies the Heart. Excellent for emotional causes of morning sickness.
HT 5 - Calms the Mind & the pulse.
BL 15 - (Heart Back Shu Point) Tonifies & Nourishes the Heart. Calms the Spirit. Clears Heart Fire.

4. Heartburn

Heartburn in often experienced during the second trimester. It is related to both the physical changes of the abdominal area and Stomach meridian issues, usually Heat. Recommendations include eating smaller meals, avoiding coffee and chocolate, limiting fluid intake when eating, avoiding spicy, fried and fatty foods. It can also be helpful to prop up the top of the body when sleeping.

Treatment is similar for all patterns. Possible variations of this condition include.
- **Stomach Heat**
- **Retention of Food in the Stomach**
- **Deficient Stomach Qi**

Signs & Symptoms
- Scanty vaginal bleeding
- Lumbar soreness
- Dizziness
- Fatigue
- Frequent urination

Tx: Tonify Stomach & Spleen. Relieve stagnation of the middle burner, Clear heat

Possible Acupuncture Points
Tradition advises against needling the Heart Meridian from around the 12th week.

Ren 12 (Stomach Mu Point) – Clears Stomach Heat. Harmonizes the Middle Burner. Descends rebellious Stomach Qi. Food Stagnation, Difficult digestion. Heartburn. Acid reflux.

Ren 14 (Heart Mu Point) - Clears Stomach Heat. Harmonizes the Middle Burner. Descends rebellious Stomach Qi. Treats heartburn.

ST 21 & ST 44 – Excellent combination to clear Stomach Heat. Alleviates pain, heartburn, & acid reflux.

LI 11 - Clears Heat. Improves down-bearing effect of Stomach Qi.

ST 36 - Tonify Qi (Spleen & Stomach). Transforms Dampness.

ST 19, ST 21, ST 34, KID 21, Ren 13 – Reduces an excess Stomach/Spleen problem.

St 36, PC 6 & Ren 12 – Combined treat Stomach & Spleen Qi Deficiency.

5. Constipation

Blood or Qi Deficiency can dry the intestines and cause constipation. Qi stagnation is also possible during the first trimester as the fetus is growing and the abdomen is changing.

5.1 Blood Deficiency

Signs & Symptoms
- Difficult, dry stools
- Pale complexion
- Blurred vision
- Tired
- Possibly depressed

Tongue: Pale, thin
Pulse: Choppy
Tx: Nourish Blood, moisten intestines & tonify Liver

Possible Acupuncture Points
ST 36 - Tonify Qi & Blood
BL 17 (Diaphragm Shu) - Hui meeting point of the Blood, Builds Blood
Liv 8 - Tonify Liver & Blood

5.2 Kidney Yang Deficiency

Signs & Symptoms
- Difficult bowel movements with tiredness afterwards
- Sore back
- Sensations of cold
- Frequent, pale urine
Tongue: Pale, wet
Pulse: Deep, weak
Tx: Tonify Kidney Yang. Warm Lower Burner. Moisten Intestines.

Possible Acupuncture Points
ST 36 with moxa - Tonify Qi
BL 23 (Kidney Shu) – Tonifies Yang Qi & builds Blood
BL 25 (Large Intestine Shu) – Moves the stools in the bowels. For constipation from Qi Deficiency.
Kid 7 - Tonify Kidney Yang

5.3 Kidney Yin Deficiency

Signs & Symptoms
- Dry stools
- Thirst with little desire to drink
- Dry mouth usually worse in the evening
- Sore back and/or knees
- Tinnitus
- Night sweats
Tongue: Red with no coat
Pulse: Floating, empty
Tx: Tonify Yin, Moisten Intestines

Possible Acupuncture Points
ST 36 - Tonifies Qi & Blood. Moves stools.
Kid 3 - Tonifies Kidney Yin
Kid 6 - Tonifies Kidney Yin

BL 23 (Kidney Shu) – Tonifies the Kidneys & builds Blood
BL 25 (Large Intestine Shu) – Moves stools in the bowels. For constipation from Qi Deficiency

5.4 Qi Stagnation

Signs & Symptoms
- Pebbly stools
- Belching
- Irritability
- Abdominal distention
Tongue: May be normal, darkish or slightly red on sides.
Pulse: Wiry
Tx: Regulate Liver. Move Stagnation.

Possible Acupuncture Points
Liv 3 – Regulates the Liver, Moves Qi
Ren 10 – Aids the Stomach - 1st three months only
GB 34 – Regulates the Liver. Moves stagnation.
Liv 2, Liv 3 – Clears Heat & Liver Qi Stagnation. Only use Liv 2 if lots of heat.

6. Hemorrhoids

Hemorrhoids may arise from the changes in vasculature due to pregnancy. Qi deficiencies can bring about weakness (prolapses). Constipation and prolonged labor can lead to hemorrhoids. Possible variations include:

- **Blood Deficiency**
- **Heat in the Blood**
- **Blood Stasis**
- **Qi Stagnation**
- **Damp Heat**

Tx: Clear hemorrhoids & pathogenic factors. Treatment is similar for all patterns.

Possible Acupuncture Points
BL 57, BL 58 – Specific for Hemorrhoids (Divergent channel winds around anal region)
DU 20 – Raises sinking Qi
Erbai (EX Point – Two Whites) – Prolapse of the rectum & hemorrhoids.

If the patient has a history of miscarriages or has undergone IVF avoid needling distal leg points. May add additional points to move Qi Stagnation and clear Blood Heat.

7. Breech Baby

A breech baby's head points upwards and therefore the baby is likely to come out feet first. Breech presentations affect 4% of pregnancies but most of the time the baby turns by the 36th week. If the baby continues to be breech most doctors advise a C-section.

Clinical trials indicate that acupuncture and moxibustion have a success rate of anywhere between 69% and 85% in turning the baby. The best results are obtained between weeks 32 and 35. After week 37 the baby may be too tightly wedged to move.

During treatment, the patient is semi seated with the upper body at a 45-degree angle to facilitate breathing. A moxa stick is used to activate **BL 67** on both feet for 15 minutes. Continue treatment for 10 days at a minimum of 2 treatments day. The moxa should feel relaxing, warm, and not too hot. The patient and her partner can be trained to do the treatment at home for 15 minutes twice a day.

Only insert **needles with or without moxa at BL 67** after 37 weeks. Far Infrared Light can be used to warm the feet. Other issues such as a twisted hip can be treated at the same time.

It is believed that the treatment creates more space in the Uterus in which the baby can turn if it wishes to do so. During the treatment, the baby may move more than usual because of the sensation of increased space.

If the patient feels the baby turn, she should stop the treatment and ask her medical doctor or midwife to check the baby's position.

If there is a physical obstruction limiting the movement of the baby such as fibroids, placement of the placenta and umbilical cord, treatment may have no effect.

A pregnant woman should **not** try to turn a breech baby:

- If she has twins
- If she has had a previous caesarean section
- If she experienced bleeding during pregnancy
- If she suffers from high blood pressure or gestational diabetes.

Postpartum Depression

Postpartum Depression is depression suffered by a mother following childbirth, typically arising from the combination of hormonal changes, psychological adjustment to motherhood, and fatigue. Postpartum depression's signs and symptoms include:

- Mood swings
- Unhappiness
- Insomnia or Hypersomnia
- Psychomotor retardation
- Suicidal tendencies
- Cognitive dysfunction
- Low libido
- Exhaustion
- Anger or Irritability
- Lack of appetite
- Not bonding with the baby
- Low self-esteem

In Traditional Chinese Medicine, postpartum depression may present with additional symptoms such as

- Low energy levels
- Stifling chest sensation
- Sighing
- Loss of appetite
- Dream disturbed sleep
- Frustration
- Crying
- Worry
- Sadness
- Melancholy

Acupuncture causes a significant reduction in the symptoms of depression in the short to medium term. Research indicates that acupuncture balances various neuro-transmitters, reduces the brain's reaction to stress, relaxes the stressful spirit, regulates and treats the physical symptoms, and relieves the depressive and anxious state.

From a TCM perspective, acupuncture treatment soothes the Liver, regulates Qi, strengthens the Kidneys, calms the Shen of the Heart, and clears the Brain.

Possible Acupuncture Points

DU 20 or Sishencong - The head is the gathering site of all Yang & is the house of the Mind. These points calm the Spirit, benefit the brain, lower Qi in anxiety cases & raise Qi in depression.
Liv 3 & **LI 4** - Four Gates - Both are Yuan source points. Together they regulate Qi, Blood, Yin & Yang. They also soothe the Liver & calm the Mind. **Liv 3** treats anxiety, palpitations & nervousness. Also helpful for the treatment of insomnia. **LI 4** or the Valley of Hope & Spirit, relieves anger, depression, numbness & emotional holding.
PC 6 - Luo-connecting point that benefits Heart Qi & calms the Mind. Treats insomnia, anxiety, mania, poor memory, apprehensiveness, fear, fright & sadness.
SP 6 - Meeting point of three Yin meridians of the foot. Regulates Qi & Blood. Treats insomnia & disharmony of Heart & Kidneys.
ST 36 - Benefits Stomach Qi, Yuan Qi & Blood production. Relaxes anxiety, panic attacks, mood swings, abandonment issues, depression, self-abuse & self-esteem issues, worry & codependency.

Giovanni Maciocia, world-renowned expert in Traditional Chinese Medicine, believes the treatment of depression must include the opening of the Du Mai or Governing Vessel as it originates in the Kidneys, goes through the Heart and anchors in the brain.

In addition, according to Giovanni the spiritual aspects of depression must be treated in addition to the base pattern accompanying the disorder such as Qi Stagnation, Kidney Yang Deficiency or Blood Stasis.

Long-standing chronic emotions can lead to Qi Stagnation which can occur in any organ. In the context of emotional problems Qi Stagnation of the Heart and Lungs is common.

Sadness and grief can lead to Qi Deficiency which can evolve into Qi Stagnation of the Heart and Lungs. Worry can lead to Qi Stagnation of the Spleen, Lungs and Heart. Worry and anger can lead to Qi Rising. Guilt affects the Heart and Kidneys and restrains the movement of the Hun (Spirit of the Liver).

Diet that leads to Blood Deficiency or Phlegm can be a factor in depression. Phlegm is very often a factor in chronic depression.

Points to Open the Du Mai

SI 3 & BL 62 – Opens Du Mai. (**SI 3** also for Mania Depression)

Plus one of the following:
DU 11 - Nourishes the Heart & Shen. Deficiency conditions of the Heart. Brings Yang Qi to the Heart. Calms the Spirit. Keeps you in the here and now – daily living. Treated when the Heart is lacking nourishment leading to sadness, anxiety, palpitations, timidity & shortness of breath. Trapped in a defeating state of mind unable to see the larger picture.
Du 16 (Root of the Spirit World) - For Hun coming & going too much. Mania, incessant talking, mad walking, desire to commit suicide, sadness & fear with fright palpitations. Relieves trauma, shock & nightmares.
Du 20 - Lowers Qi in anxiety cases & raises Qi in Depression. Combined with GB 40 tonifies clear Yang rising to the head.
Du 24 - Calms the Spirit. Anchors & settles anxiety. Eliminates old patterns. Treats depression, palpitations, fright, anxiety, addictions & Yang mental excess. Lowers Liver Yang. Combine with GB 13 for anxiety.
GB 13 - Prevents emotional extremes. Gathers Jing to the Brain. Works on Jing, Kidneys & Marrow. Root of the Shen. Makes Shen return to its root. Connects Shen & Jing, Heart & Kidneys.
GB 40 - Helps with decision making. Moves the Hun in & out. Activates other points. Helps the ascending of Liver Qi to the Heart & Shen allowing for the extending of the movement of relationships.

Treating the Five Spiritual Aspects of Depression

Kidneys - Zhi - Will Power-Drive

BL 23 & BL 52 - Needle even in the absence of Kidney Deficiency symptoms especially if the person is depressed for a long period of time. Governs emotional stamina & spiritual renewal. Releases fear, phobia, trauma, emotional numbness, anger, depression & withdrawal. BL 52 - Stimulates the ZHI of the Kidneys to stimulate initiative & drive on a mental level.

Du 4 - Stabilizes the Kidneys. Clears the Brain. Calms the Spirit. Source of Essence. Relieves disorientation, forgetfulness, fear, terror & nightmares.

Kid 3 - Balances the Kidneys, strengthens will power & the Brain. Treats fear. Stabilizes intimate relationships. Relieves feelings of abandonment, guilt. Treats issues emanating from incest.

Liver - Hun - Ethereal Soul - Anger-Irritability

The Hun is not coming and going as it should. Creates a lack of sense of direction. In Bi Polar cases the Phlegm is blocking the coming and going of the Hum. Creates either an excess of movement or a deficiency of the movement of the Hun.

Emotional stress resulting from anger, worry, guilt, shame, sadness and grief affect both the Heart and the Liver. This restrains the movement of the Hun. If the pulse is not wiry, anger or suppressed anger is not a cause of depression.

GB 40 - Helps with decision making. Moves the Hun in and out. Activates other points. Helps the ascending of Liver Qi to the Heart & Shen allowing for the extending of the movement of relationships.

BL 47 (Outer Bladder Line) - Gate of Ethereal Soul - Point of spiritual aspect or Hun of the Liver. Regulates the movement of the Hun in both depression and mania.

Heart - Shen - Sadness

Du 24 - Very important point. Calms the Spirit. Anchors & settles anxiety. Eliminates old patterns. Treats depression, palpitations, fright, anxiety, addictions & Yang mental excess. Lowers Liver Yang. Combine with GB 13 for anxiety.

REN 15 (Spirit Storehouse - Ren Luo Connecting Point) – Regulates the Heart. Unbinds the chest & calms the Spirit. Softens controlling personalities. Heals addictions linked to escapism (sexuality) & comfort foods.

HT 7 - Spirit gate – Yuan Source Sedation Point – Tonifies the Heart. Promotes clarity of Mind. Relaxes the Mind & body. Regulates extremes of the Heart, ups & downs. Treats insomnia, chronic stress, nervousness, mania, annoyance & depression. Relieves sadness & anxiety.

Lungs - Po - Physical Soul related to morbid thoughts of death.

Du 24 - Very important point. Calms the Spirit. Eliminates old patterns. Treats depression, anxiety, addictions & Yang mental excess. Lowers Liver Yang. Combine with GB 13 for anxiety.
Lu 7 - Sadness. Poor memory. Propensity to laughter.
BL 13 or DU 12 or BL 42 – Related to the Lungs. All these points have to do with thoughts of death.

Spleen - Yi - Intellect - Obsessive thinking or thoughts.

DU 24 - Very important point. Calms the Spirit. Anchors & settles anxiety. Eliminates old patterns. Treats depression, palpitations, fright, anxiety, addictions & Yang mental excess. Lowers Liver Yang. Combine with GB 13 for anxiety.
GB 13 - Prevents emotional extremes. Gathers Jing to the Brain. Works on Jing, Kidneys & Marrow. Root of the Shen. Makes Shen return to its root. Connects Shen & Jing, Heart & Kidneys.
DU 20 - Lowers Qi in anxiety cases & raises Qi in Depression. Combined with GB 40 tonifies clear Yang rising to the head.
BL 49 – Shelter of Yi

Triple Warmer (Pericardium) - Relationship problems.

SJ 5 - For emotional projection. Reduces vulnerability. Relieves depression, sadness, withdrawal & grief.
PC 6 - Regulates the Heart & calms the Spirit. Relieves nausea, anxiety, racing heartbeat. Treats insomnia, mania, fright, sadness, fear & apprehension.
PC 7 - Clears Heat from the Heart. Treats mania, manic raving, ceaseless laughter, agitation, sadness, fright & fear, & weeping with grief.
Ren 17 (Sea of Tranquility) **-** Balances the emotions & calms the Spirit. Best point for relief of a panic attack. Treats nervousness, grief, sadness, anguish, emotional trauma, depression & hysteria.

Gall Bladder - Indecisiveness - Lack of courage.

GB 40 - Helps with decision making. Moves the Hun in & out. Activates other points. Helps the ascending of Liver Qi to the Heart & Shen allowing for the extending of the movement of relationships.
GB 13 - Prevents emotional extremes. Gathers Jing to the Brain.

Works on Jing, Kidneys & Marrow. Root of the Shen. Makes Shen return to its root. Connects Shen & Jing, Heart & Kidneys.
DU 20 - Lowers Qi in anxiety cases & raises Qi in Depression. Combined with GB 40 tonifies clear Yang rising to the head.

Additional Points:
Yin Tang (Mid-Eyebrow Point) - Spiritual & emotional healing point. Calms the Spirit, Relieves anxiety, nervousness, depression & anger. Heals trauma. Strengthens intuition.
Tai Yang - Calms the Spirit & Clears the Mind
HT 7 & SI 7 - HE 7 is the principal point on the Heart Channel to Calm & regulate the Spirit. SI 7 complements this action by treating pyscho-emotional disorders.
HT 7, BL 15, ST 41, PE 7 – Weeping with grief.
Ren 4/Ren 5/Ren 6 - Develop emotional stability. Deepen spiritual awareness. Strengthen sense of self. Treats self-abuse, addictions & codependency issues.
REN 12/Ren 13 - Hold overall body tension & stress. Release stored emotional pain related to abandonment, self-esteem, & boundary issues, anger, shame, gilt & codependency.
ST 40 - Opens the chest & Heart. Reduces Qi stagnation of Lung & Heart. Calms the Shen. Treats the Stomach & Bi Polar disorder, mania-depression, mad laughter, great happiness, desires to ascend to high places & sing, discards clothing & runs around, seeing ghosts. Works well with PC 6.
LU 1 (Letting Go) - Opens the Spirit. Release anxiety, repressed emotions, emotional holding, expectations, depression, grief, sadness & anger.
LU 3 - Window of Heaven Point – Stimulates the rising & descending of Qi. Treats Lung & Heart Qi Stagnation & mental emotional issues. Clears thoughts. Good for forgetfulness, melancholy, crying, ghost talk, sadness & weeping.
GB 20 (Gates of Consciousness) - Heals traumatic experiences. Heightens spirituality. Balances jealousy, resentment, irritability, addictions, guilt, numbness, anger & judgement.

According to the Health Medicine Institute research indicates that electroacupuncture can have positive effects in treating depression by modifying or regulating the expression of various genes related to depression. Electroacupuncture can be applied to the following acupuncture points:

DU 23 & DU 24 - Yin Tang
One acupuncture needle is inserted obliquely 0.5 to 1 cun from Yin Tang towards DU 23 / DU 24, and another needle is inserted from DU 24 penetrating DU 23 towards Yin Tang. Rotate the needles to obtain the sensation of De Qi. Then the two needles are attached to electrical current to stimulate the area between DU 23 / DU 24 & Yin Tang. The electric current stimulates the higher prefrontal regions, regulating the neural activity of fear and anxiety.

Tai Yang - GB 8 & GB 9
One acupuncture needle is inserted obliquely 0.5 to 1 cun from Tai Yang towards GB 8 /GB 9 and another needle is inserted from GB 9 penetrating GB 8 towards Tai Yang. These two needles are attached to electrical current to stimulate the area between Tai Yang and GB 8 / GB 9. The electric current stimulates the amygdala and hippocampus regions to regulate neural activity of fear and anxiety.

For both treatments apply high frequency continuous electric waves for 30 minutes once to twice a week for 6 weeks. Reevaluate after 12 visits to determine if further treatment is necessary.

Auricular Therapy

Stimulating certain ear acupoints can help patients relax, and combined with body acupuncture, can reduce symptoms in patients with minor depression, chronic anxiety disorders and general anxiety disorders. The major auricular points used for the treatment of anxiety are:

Shen Men; Point Zero & Sympathetic Autonomic Point

Press needles may be left in the ears for a minimum of 48 hours. Self-managing ASP needles can be left until they fall out on their own.

InVitro Fertilization (IVF) / Intrauterine Insemination (IUI)

Acupuncture treatments are provided in the months leading up to and immediately before and after an Insemination (IUI) or Invitro Fertilization (IVF). Caution must be observed after the procedure to avoid provoking a miscarriage.

When providing acupuncture for IVF or IUI there are three phases to treatment:
- Before IVF or IUI
- During IVF or IUI
- After IVF or IUI

Before IVF or IUI it is appropriate to treat patients for three to four months before progressing to IUI or IVF. People over 40 or with low ovarian reserve may need treatment for a longer period.

Treatment at the **pre-stage** focuses on:
- Improving general health
- Increasing Blood supply to the reproductive organs
- Improving the lining of the Uterus
- Improving egg production and egg quality
- Correcting menstrual cycle irregularities
- Addressing nutritional and lifestyle concerns
- Addressing any specific health issues that affect fertility
- Managing stress

During IVF or IUI acupuncture is performed immediately before and after the procedure to help with the implantation or insemination by reducing stress and creating a receptive environment for pregnancy. Acupuncture treatments can address any specific issues than may arise from the procedure such as abdominal pain or emotional stress.

After IVF or IUI weekly acupuncture and Chinese herbs will be necessary for up to three months after the onset of pregnancy.

This treatment helps:
- Prevent a miscarriage and an ectopic pregnancy
- Encourage the growth of the developing foetus

If supplementation or herbs are prescribed before IVF or IUI beginning early is best as they take time to work. Even if patients decide to wait to start acupuncture, they should not wait to start herbal medicine or supplementation. Taking a herbal formula 3 to 4 month prior to conception or transfer, allows the eggs to grow and mature in a nutrient rich environment.

Normally herbal medicine is discontinued during the period leading up to IUI or IVF when fertility medications are being administered by the patient's medical doctor to help improve chances of a successful pregnancy. Hormonal treatments prescribed by the medical doctor aim to increase the number of eggs that attain maturity and time the release of these eggs with their retrieval or artificial insemination, whereas herbal medicine reinforces the body's natural reproductive rhyme.

For the best interest of the patient, practitioners specialised in herbal medicine should avoid any real or perceived complications from the application of these two different and possibly contradictory treatment strategies when fertility medications are being administered during the IVF or IUI procedure.

It is important to note that IUI may or may not include hormonal therapy. Some Medical Doctors follow the natural rhythm of the patient's menstrual cycle when performing IUI.

Acupuncture as a Support to IVF

Before seeking medical reproductive assistance, it is wise for women to do everything possible to optimize their reproductive and hormonal health. A women's best response to any ART procedure depends on the proper functioning of the endocrine system a few months preceding the procedure.

Therefore, when providing acupuncture treatment to women undergoing InVitro Fertilization, for the best outcome it is preferable to start weekly treatments three months before the IVF procedure. The frequency of treatments may increase closer to the procedure or to address specific conditions that may hinder fertility.

The timing of an acupuncture treatment in relation to the menstrual cycle is of great importance. Weekly treatments follow the rhythm of the menstrual cycle. An acupuncture treatment administered between day six and eight of the stimulated menstrual cycle is optimal. In addition, if possible, it is ideal to have two acupuncture treatments on the day before or day of embryo transfer.

Before Embryo Transfer

The treatment will improve Blood flow to the Uterus and ovaries, providing a nourishing environment for the embryo by triggering vasodilation and Uterine Blood flow. It also helps minimize cramping and relaxes both the cervix and the Mind. Pre-transfer acupuncture points of high priority are **SP 8, SP 10, Liv 3, ST 29** and **Ren 4.**

SP 8 - Tonifies & invigorates Blood. Transforms Dampness. Regulates the Uterus. Minimizes Uterine cramping in preparation for transfer.
SP 10 - Leads Blood from the "Sea of Blood" to the Uterus
Liv 3 - Moves Q & removes Stagnation. Invigorates Blood. Lowers Liver Yang. Calms the Spirit.
ST 29 - Returns Blood to the Uterus. Reduces inflammation of the ovaries & fallopian tubes.
Ren 4 - Reinforces Kidney Yin & Yang & warms the Uterus via the Ren Meridian (the source of the Essence of the body)
Zi Gong - Brings Qi & Blood to the Uterus
Ren 6 - (Sea of Qi) Tonifies the Kidneys, Spleen & Original Qi. Invigorates the Blood.
SP 6 - Crossing point of the Liver, Spleen & Kidney meridians. Promotes Uterine Blood circulation to prepare a Yin environment for the baby. Research shows that strong stimulate of this point can make the Uterus contract which brings Blood to the endometrium.
DU 20 - Calms the Spirit. Uplifts the Qi to support implantation.
PC 6 - Calms the Mind. Clears Heat. Reduces Blood pressure. Promotes the opening & relaxation of the cervix.

After Embryo Transfer

Acupuncture treatments after embryo transfer should start as soon as possible. After the embryo has been implanted acupuncture helps calm the Uterus and avoid contractions which could expel the embryo. Post-transfer points include **Du 20, Kid 3, BL 57 & SP 6, and PC 6**.

IVF patients need very special care in the first twelve weeks of pregnancy, including Kidney Yin and Yang tonics. After embryo implantation, herbal formulas can be prescribed to reduce the risk of miscarriage, and treat issues such as anemia, fatigue, nausea, severe vomiting, and threatened miscarriage.

DU 20 - Calms the Shen & lifts the Qi
Sishencong (Four points around Du 20) - Calms the Mind avoiding contraction of the Uterus
Kid 3 - Tonifies Essence & nourishes the Kidneys
BL 57 - Relaxes sinews & moves Blood. Often combined with **Sp 6** to improve Blood flow to the ovaries & Uterus.
PC 6 - This is THE point for nausea & vomiting. It is also one of the most relaxing acupuncture points & is used for both insomnia and anxiety. Calms the Mind. Harmonizes the Stomach. Clears Heat. Reduces Blood pressure.
HT 7 - Calms the Mind to avoid Uterus contraction
Ren 4 - Reinforce Kidney Yin & Yang. Warms the Uterus.
ST 36 (Often combined with **Li 4**) – Increases energy levels by strengthening the overall constitution. Builds Blood & Qi, resolves edema & harmonizes the meridians that control the digestive functions. Holds the Qi preventing Qi collapse which could lead to a miscarriage. Strengthens the Spleen & Stomach Qi. Great point for diarrhea, constipation, gastric pain & indigestion. The Large Intestine & Uterus all belong to the smooth muscle group, so diarrhea can cause a miscarriage. Regulates Qi & Blood to help prevent cramping.
Li 4 – Moves Qi. Minimizes pain & circulates Qi in the Uterus to help prevent cramping & reduce the movement of the fetus in the Uterus. This point is Counter Indicated in Pregnancy & can be used to abort a dead fetus. But it can be used here as the embryo is not yet implanted so there is no pregnancy.
SP 10 - Leads Blood from the "Sea of Blood" to the Uterus. Helps prevent cramping.

Auricular Acupuncture

Left Ear	Right Ear
Shenmen – Relaxation & analgesic effects	Uterus – Supports the Uterus
Brain Points – Regulates the endocrine system.	Endocrine Points – Supports the body's endocrinological functions

Acupuncture as a Support to IUI

Success rates for IUI (Intrauterine Insemination) have been determined to be from 15 to 20%. Acupuncture and Chinese Medicine can greatly improve these success rates. Acupuncture treatments differ somewhat from the treatment protocols for Invitro Fertilization.

With IUI the sperm is introduced into the Uterus at the optimal time to meet with the women's egg. Hormonal treatments are often used to increase the number of eggs and to time the release of the eggs from the follicles with the introduction of the sperm.

Avoid herbal medicine if hormones are used to influence the menstrual cycle and release of the eggs so as not to conflict with the treatment the patient is receiving from her medical doctor. The fertility drugs introduced by the medical doctor work to control the menstrual cycle contrary to herbal medicine which supports and reinforces the women's natural cycle.

Acupuncture treatments should proceed as usual following the four phases of the menstrual cycle. Consideration may be given to increasing the number of treatments before and after artificial insemination to support the process and address any issues that may arise such as increased levels of stress resulting from the medical procedure.

Also after insemination by the Doctor, do not treat aggressively to avoid disrupting the natural process of implantation of the fertilized ovum into the endometrium.

Acupuncture Induction

Acupuncture induction can be very helpful in supporting the birthing process. It has been utilized in China to successfully induce overdue labor since the Jin Dynasty (AD 265 - 420). When applied under the appropriate circumstances, it is a safe and powerful method to facilitate the delivery process.

Research indicates that acupuncture successfully:
- Prepares the uterus and cervix for labor
- Initiates the onset of labor
- Reduces the pain of contractions
- Shortens the average time of labor
- Reduces recovery time
- Significantly decreases the need for medical intervention
(Smith 2004, Betts 2006).

A clinical study in New Zealand (Betts & Lennox, 2006) showed that giving women pre-birth acupuncture resulted in a:

- 35% reduction in medical inductions (43% reduction in women having their first baby)
- 31% reduction in the epidurals
- 32% reduction in emergency caesarean delivery
- 9% increase in normal vaginal births

Acupuncture for the induction of labor is a very gentle process and is less of a jolt to the system than drugs which tend to react very quickly. Therefore, it is wise use it first but always with the approval of the patient's medical team. This procedure should only be initiated once the baby is mature and low in the abdomen, between 38 and 41 weeks into the pregnancy.

The first thing a woman should establish is the accuracy of her due date. The due date is based on a woman having a 28-day menstrual cycle, ovulating on day 14. If the cycle is longer, for example 35 days with ovulation occurring on day 21, then the due date would be 7 days later. Furthermore, medical professionals believe that generally a woman can safely go 10 days past her due date.

When deciding whether to induce the baby, it is important to respect both the needs of the baby and the women's body. If the cervix is not ripe, an induction can cause ineffective contractions that can lead to a long, difficult labor. Cervical ripening is when the cervix softens and stretches promoting its dilation in preparation for the birth of the child.

Pregnant women can opt for cervical ripening treatments between week 37 and week 41 of pregnancy. Research has shown that acupuncture for cervical ripening lessens the need for medical induction, epidurals and emergency cesareans while hastening the delivery time. **Spleen 6** and **Large Intestine 4** are the two major acupuncture points used in this procedure.

For the induction to be successful, the cervix needs to be dilated by at least 2 cm and the baby's head should be engaged in the pelvis. A premature induction can lead to problems for both the baby and the mother. Acupuncture is very effective in stimulating the uterus. But if the timing of the induction is off the mother can be up all-night with contractions, anticipating labor, just to see the contractors subside.

When the time comes for labor, the mother could be physically and emotionally drained. Hyper contractions can also affect the baby's heart rate and breathing, making a vaginal delivery more challenging.

If the cervix is ripe and the patient is past her due date, not in early labor, and the baby and placenta and amniotic fluid levels are within normal limits, acupuncture with the health care provider's consent is an effective way to start labor especially if the patient commits to daily sessions and allows adequate time for treatment.

Women will often progress into labour after their first treatment, but more commonly after two to three treatments. Rarely acupuncture induction may require four treatments. If a woman is showing signs of pre-labour rumblings such as cramping, lower back pain, a mild downward bearing sensation or diffuse abdominal tightening, it is highly likely that she will quickly progress into labour.

Each treatment may take up to 1.5 hours. The couple should come to the clinic prepared to go to the hospital or birthing place if the contractions appear at regular five-minute intervals or less.

The patient is seated comfortably on a chair or a treatment table. The needles are applied bilaterally stimulating in stages waiting between each stage to determine if the contractions come more regularly.

Some women will have little sensation during the treatment while others experience downward movement, urinary urge and abdominal tightening during and up to 5 hours after treatment. Woman should go straight home after treatment, remain quiet and allow the body to rest in preparation for labor.

Start with inserting a needle at **BL 67** bilaterally, manually stimulating the points manually and observing how the patient responds. This point stimulates uterine contractions and can also turn the fetus. They are located on the little toes, near the outer edge of the nail.

Progress to **SP 6** (Black Lead) and **ST 36** (Red Lead) bilaterally, stimulating with electro acupuncture or manually as before for 5 to 10 minutes. Look for contractions and hardening of the mother's abdomen.

SP 6 - Promotes the ripening of the cervix. Strong stimulate of this point makes the Uterus contract.
ST 36 - Hastens delivery and increases energy levels. Treats anxiety, depression, panic attacks and mood swings.

Another option is to needle **Ren 4** and **SP 6** together with electrostimulation on SP 6 to open the cervix, encourage the descent of the baby and increase contractions. Care should be taken when needling Ren 4 to avoid puncturing the amniotic sac.

Add **BL 31** and **BL 32** bilaterally to relieve back pain and stimulate the muscles of the Uterus, needling to the foramen with at least 50 mm length needles with the client seated or sideling. Stimulate the needles with either electro acupuncture or manually. Do for 5 to 10 minutes, once again looking for contraction and hardening of the mother's abdomen.

It is important to check the abdomen for contractions with the palm as the mother may not necessarily be aware of the increased frequency of contractions.

Adding **Liv 3** (Black Lead) and **LI 4** (Red Lead), known as the four gates, can really move things along. Together they vigorously activate Qi and Blood ensuring their free and smooth passage throughout the body.

Liv 3 - Major point to activate the Chong Mai. Relieves stress, tension, anxiety and insomnia that may contribute to the failure to start labor. Also helpful for relieving lower back pain during labor.
LI 4 - Helps the woman push downwards and stimulates uterine contractions.

ST 44 – Helps reduce pain experienced by the patient.

Add auricular points such as Shenmen, Uterus, Endocrine and other points for body areas experiencing discomfort.

Other Possible Points

PC 8 - Considered by some to be very useful in inducing labor.
Kid 1 - Helps pull the energy downward and reduces the stress and anxiety of the mother.
BL 60 - Promotes labor, eases labor pain and reduces obstruction. May encourage the baby to descend in the early stages of labor.
GB 21 - Promotes the downward flow of energy and will stimulate contractions encouraging the baby to descend into the pelvic and engage either before labor for the first born or during labor for the second or later births. It also provides relief from labor pain.

Chinese Herbal Medicine

Chinese Herbal Medicine can be safely utilized to induce labor. The herbs move and invigorate Blood to awaken and dislodge the fetus, descend energy, and nourish Blood to help dilate the cervix. Women should commence herbal induction treatment up to 4 days in advance of a scheduled medical induction.

Shortly after consuming the herbal medicine it is common for women to experience lower abdominal tightening and sensations ranging from mild cramping to sharper, stabbing period-like vaginal pain. This is a good sign that the formula is having an effect and that labor is imminent.

Endometriosis

Endometriosis is caused by the implantation of fibrous connective tissue in the peritoneal cavity causing inflammation and painful periods. It is largely a disease of young women (25 to 40 years old) and is a major cause of infertility. Twenty to 40% of women with infertility issues and 25% of women using IVF suffer from endometriosis. In fact, endometriosis and Polycystic Ovarian Syndrome combined account for a large part of infertility issues.

Endometrial tissue is normally confined to the lining of the Uterus. With endometriosis it grows into the uterine muscles or elsewhere in the pelvic/abdominal cavity, such as in the fallopian tubes, around the ovaries, uterine ligaments, bladder and intestines. The most common location of endometriosis lesions is around the ovaries.

The endometrial tissue bleeds cyclically in response to the woman's menstrual cycle. The Blood has no way of leaving the body, so it stagnates at the site of the endometrial implantation. This can cause painful pelvic cavity inflammation, adhesions and scaring.

Both Western and Chinese medicine believe that endometriosis occurs when menstrual Blood is pushed back into the Uterus due to the wearing of tampons, the insertion of Intrauterine Devices (IUD), or practicing intercourse during menses. Uterine abnormalities such as cervical stenosis or congenital pelvic defects can also contribute to this disorder.

Menstrual Blood contains fragments of endometrial tissue. Therefore, the tubal reflux that results from the blockage of menstrual Blood may lead to the implantation of endometrial tissue in the pelvic structures.

Diagnosis of endometriosis is complicated by the fact that symptoms are very similar to other diseases such as Pelvic Inflammatory Disease, Ovarian Tumors and Irritable Bowel Syndrome. About 40% of women diagnosed with endometriosis report no symptoms other than infertility. The major symptom of endometrioses is painful periods or dysmenorrhea sometimes accompanied by nausea and vomiting. Other symptoms include:

- Heavy periods or irregular bleeding
- Fatigue
- Diarrhea
- Dyspareunia or difficult or painful sexual intercourse
- Dizziness or headaches with periods

Women with endometriosis or fibroids often experience a sediment - like menstrual flow with dark, brown, clotted Blood that has oxidized.

According to Randine Lewis, author of the Infertility Cure, static Blood may trigger an immune response to the increased toxicity in the form of inflammation to protect the body from the endometrial cells growing outside the Uterus.

When the immune system is unable to eradicate the endometrial tissue, it reacts to all the misplaced tissue creating a toxic environment for an implanting embryo. This condition is often characterised by TCM as Blood Stasis with excess Heat or Damp Heat. Treatment for resolving the immune system response it so clear internal Blood Heat and calm the Uterus with acupuncture and herbs.

As mentioned above, the main cause of endometriosis is Blood Stasis. The specific pathology is Blood moving out of its original place in the blood vessels and stagnating in the Chong and Ren Meridians. Therefore, Blood cannot arrive on time for menses and period disorders occur. The Uterus meridians are blocked therefore patients suffer from irregular and painful periods, and infertility.

Western hormonal treatments for endometriosis are designed to stop ovulation by reducing the levels of estrogen. Unfortunately, once the treatment is discontinued the condition returns. Endometriosis resolves during pregnancy due to the lack of periods. After pregnancy endometriosis returns but often with a marked regression of lesions.

Laparoscopy is the most common procedure used to diagnose and remove mild to moderate endometriosis. Doctors may revert to surgery for the treatment of severe endometriosis that can't be treated with laparoscopy. After surgery, the toxic effects of lingering endometrial cells can continue to contaminate fallopian tubes affecting the egg's ability to become fertilized as it travels towards the uterus.

Chinese Medicine identifies several causes of endometrioses which lead to the retention of menses or scanty periods (menstrual Blood not flowing down during the period).

- Early sexual activity which damages the Chong and Ren vessels, causing Blood Stasis.
- Invasion of the Uterus by external Cold, which contracts the Uterus causing Blood to stagnate. This condition is worse before, during and just after the period, during puberty and just after childbirth. This is the most common cause of Blood Stasis in teenagers and is worsened by sitting in damp spaces or being scantly dressed during freezing temperatures.
- Intercourse during menstruation
- Excessive physical work which weakens the Chong and Ren vessels, and depletes the Kidneys and Spleen especially at puberty.
- Tampons and intra-uterine devices that block the normal downward flow of menstrual Blood leading to the retention of menses and Blood Stasis.
- Emotional issues such as anger, repressed anger, worry, shame and guilt can lead to Qi Stagnation and eventually Blood Stasis.

Acupuncture treatments help reduce painful periods and activate the Chong and Ren Vessels to increase Blood flow to the Uterus. To achieve positive results a herbal formula must be prescribe in addition to acupuncture to strongly invigorate and break Blood. Please note that herbs that invigorate and break Blood are counter indicated in pregnancy.

Practitioners must not combine Chinese herbs with Western hormonal treatment as Chinese herbs cannot regulate a woman's hormonal system when ovulation is being suppressed artificially. The objective of TCM is to regulate the hormones and the menstrual cycle and eliminate Blood Stasis. This can not be achieved if the patient is taking medication to stop ovulation.

Blood Stasis is always present in endometriosis, but other mainly deficiency patterns are also present. Nevertheless, the focus of treatment is always Blood stasis especially if the periods are painful. Painful periods with large dark clots are a definite sign of Blood Stasis.

Additional critical signs are retention of menses or insufficient discharge of Blood during menses.

The tongue presentation is often normal if the Blood Stasis is not severe or if the condition has just appeared recently. As the condition worsens purple sublingual veins will appear, followed by a purple color along the sides of the tongue in the Uterus area. In severe chronic cases the whole tongue will become purple.

The root cause of the disorder is Kidney Yang Deficiency which is mainly the result of external Cold that can lead to luteal insufficiency. Kidney Yang Deficiency is more common than Kidney Yin Deficiency as a cause of endometriosis. Kidney Deficiency may occur with a disharmony of the Liver and Spleen. Other patterns related to this disorder are Blood Deficiency, Heat Coagulating, and Dampness or Phlegm blockage.

Kidney Yang Deficiency prevents the body temperature from rising after ovulation. Blood Stasis prevents the body temperature from dropping during the period.

The treatment of endometriosis can be viewed as supporting the downward and outward flow of menstrual Blood. Women experiencing this condition can do breathing exercises during menses that move Qi downward and use pads or menstrual cups instead of tampons.

World-renowned acupuncturist, Giovanni Marciocia, recommends treating endometriosis according to the Four Phases of the menstrual cycle as it benefits both the symptoms and the root cause of the disorder. According to this treatment approach, the Blood is invigorated in phases one and four, moderating the treatment in phase one if the periods are heavy, and the Kidneys are reinforced in phases two and three.

In addition to regulating the menses according to the Four Phases, the treatment objective is to move the Qi downward to stop pain, calm the Heart which has an important influence on Blood, invigorate and break Blood, and supplement the Kidneys. Breaking Blood can only be achieved with the use of an appropriate herbal formula.

It is important to warm the Uterus in phases three and four even in the absence of Cold signs in order to ensure the growth of Yang Qi unless there are signs of Liver Fire or Damp Heat.

Opening the Ren and Chong Meridians is essential in the treatment of painful periods and endometriosis. Both meridians treat the Uterus, regulate menses and resolve masses. The Chong Mai or Sea of Blood is used to move Blood. The Ren Mai regulates the period and menstruation. It tonifies the Kidneys and promotes ovulation and fertility. Activate the Chong Mai in phases one and four and the Ren Mai in phases two and three coupled with other points such as Ren 4.

To activate these special meridians needle Spleen 4 on the right side and Pericardium 6 on the left for the Chong Mai, and Lung 7 on the right and Kidney 6 on the left for the Ren Mai. Leave for 10 minutes before adding additional needles.

Main Treatment Points:

Chong Mai: SP 4 & PC 6, Kid 14, SP 10, Liv 3, ST 30
Moves Blood in the Chong Mai and Uterus - Important in Phases 1 & 4

Ren Mai: Lu 7 & Kid 6, Ren 4, St 28, St 29, Zi Gong
Regulates period & tonifies the Kidneys - Important in Phases 2 & 3
(ST 29 & Zi Gong move Qi in the ovaries & fallopian tubs)

Du Mai Si 3 & BL 62, Ren 4
Can use instead of Ren Mai if Kidney Yang is Deficient

Points According to Pattern:

Blood Stasis: SP 10, Kid 14, PC 6, BL 17, SP 6, Liv 3
Damp Phlegm: SP 9, SP 6, Ren 9, ST 28, BL 22, ST 40, Ren 5
Kidney Yang Deficiency: Kid 3, ST 36, BL 23, BL 20, Ren 4

ST 28 & ST 29, SP 12 & SP 13, Kid 14 – Move Qi & Blood locally
(During the Menstrual Phase chose points according to areas of pain or where masses can be palpated)

It takes a minimum of one to two years of treatments to resolve endometriosis. Positive changes in heath will appear earlier such as less painful periods, longer cervical secretions, more regular periods, less headaches, a more stable temperature chart and a more normal tongue color. A key sign of progress is the reduction of premenstrual spotting which reflects a reduction in the amount of stagnant Blood remaining inside the pelvis.

According to Giovanni Marciocia two of the major patterns involve in endometriosis are:
1. Blood Stasis from Kidney Yang Deficiency & Dampness
2. Blood Stasis from Stagnation of Cold in the Uterus, Kidney Yang Deficiency & Dampness

1. Blood Stasis from Kidney Yang Deficiency & Dampness

Kidney Yang Deficiency Signs and Symptoms
- Dizziness
- Tinnitus
- Depression
- Feeling Cold
- Lower backache
- Painful periods
- Pale-red menstrual Blood
- Water retention and bloating before period
- Abdominal pain relieved by pressure and the application of heat
Tongue: Pale & wet
Pulse: Deep, weak

Plus:
- Mid-cycle hypogastric pain
- Scanty or heavy periods
- Dark Blood with clots
- Possible abdominal masses
- Vaginal discharge
Tongue: Swollen, pale with purple sides, sticky coating
Pulse: Deep, weak, slippery, wiry

Tx Phase 1 & 4: Invigorate Blood. Break Blood. Eliminate stasis.

Possible Acupuncture Points
SP 4 & PC 6 – Opens the Chong Mai. Moves Blood.
Ren 3, Ren 4 & Ren 6 - Use together help relieve menstrual pain.
Ren 3 - Clears stagnant Blood in the abdomen.
Ren 4 - The meeting point of the Ren & Chong Vessels. It strengthens the Kidneys, fortifies original Qi, warms the Spleen & aids in digestion. It relieves menstrual pain & assists conception by promoting the circulation of Qi & Blood. With SP 6 reinforces Kidney Yin.
Liv 3 - Moves Liver Qi & removes stagnation.
Kid 14 - Point of the Chong Mai & major point to move Blood.
ST 29 - Warms the Lower Jiao. Invigorates Blood & regulates menstruation.
SP 10 - Moves, cools & tonifies Blood. Regulates the circulation of Qi & Blood.

Herbal Formula = Modified Gui Zhi Fu Ling Wan – Cinnamon & Poria Formula (Modify formula if bleeding excessive)

Tx Phase 2 & 3: Warm and supplement Kidney Yang. Tonify Spleen.

Possible Acupuncture Points
Lu 7 & Kid 6 - Ren Mai. Tonifies the Kidneys.
Ren 4 - Meeting point of the Ren & Chong Vessels. Strengthens the Kidneys, fortifies original Qi, warms the Spleen & aids in digestion. It relieves menstrual pain & assists conception by promoting the circulation of Qi & Blood.
DU 4 - Tonifies the Kidneys. Strengthens Jing
BL 23 - Warms the Uterus. Tonifies Jing. Fortifies Kidney Yang
Kid 3 - Tonifies Jing & Kidney Yin & Yang.
ST 36 - Tonifies Original Qi. Nourishes Blood
St 28 - (Water Passage - Level with Ren 4) – Regulates body fluids. Almost exclusively used for excess patterns of obstruction.
Zi Gong – Nourishes Essence & fertility. Brings Qi & Blood to the Uterus. Treats lower abdominal pain due to obstruction of Qi & Blood.

Herbal Formula = You Gui Wan – Restore the Right Kidney Pill

The presence of Dampness if very common in endometriosis. This condition should be treated in phases 3 & 4.

Possible Acupuncture Points
SP 9 - Drains damp from the Lower Burner
Ren 9 - Expels Dampness. Tonifies the Spleen. Regulates Water Passages.
ST 28 – (Water Passage - Level with Ren 4) – Regulates body fluids. Almost exclusively used for excess patterns of obstruction. Combine with **Kid 14** a point of the Chong Mai & major point to move Blood.
ST 40 – Resolves Dampness & Phlegm

Dampness in the Uterus can be treated with acupuncture supplemented by the herbal formula Si Miao San or the Four Marvel Formula. This formula is used to treat a variety of damp-heat issues affecting the lower body.

2. Blood Stasis from Stagnation of Cold in the Uterus, Kidney Yang Deficiency & Dampness

Spasmic, strong pain with cramps and a desire for heat on the abdomen indicate Cold in the Uterus. Ask the patient if she feels cold or colder during her period. Younger women, girls and teenagers are more affected by stagnation of Cold in the Uterus.

Signs & Symptoms of Kidney Yang Deficiency plus
- Delayed periods
- Severe painful periods relieved by application of hot water bottle on tummy
- Scanty menstrual bright Blood with small, dark clots
- Feeling of fullness & heaviness
- Low back & limb pain with coldness
- Cold hands and feet
- Low libido
- Clear & profuse vaginal discharge
- Fatigue
- Possibly poor appetite, feel full easily
- Bloated Stomach
- Edema
- Loose stools

- Frequently pass clear urine
Tongue: Swollen, pale bluish or bluish purple with teeth marks & sticky white coating
Pulse: Weak, slow, tight & deep.

Tx Phase 1: Invigorate Blood. Eliminate Stasis. Scatter Cold. Warm the Uterus.
Herbal Formula = Gui Zhi Fu Ling Wan - Cinnamon & Poria Formula
Tx Phase 2: Tonify & warm Kidney Yang. Tonify Spleen Qi.
Herbal Formula = You Gui Wan - Restore the Right Kidney Pill

Tx Phase 3: Tonify warm Kidney Yang. Supplement Spleen Qi. Resolve Dampness & warm the Uterus.
Herbal Formula = You Gui Wan - Restore the Right Kidney Pill

Tx Phase 4: Invigorate Blood. Eliminate Stasis. Scatter Cold. Resolve Dampness.
Herbal Formula = Wen Jing Tang – Warm the Menses Decoction

Refer to the previous pattern for recommended acupuncture points for Blood Stasis, Kidney Yang Deficiency and Dampness.

Possible Acupuncture Points for Stagnation of Cold in the Uterus:

Moxa: Important to use Moxa when treating Blood Stasis from Cold. Ren 4 is an excellent point to treat this condition. Also consider points to tonify Spleen Qi and Kidney Yang.

SP 4 & PC 6 with Moxa on Ren 4 – Painful periods from Cold in the Uterus. Ren 4 is the meeting point of the Ren & Chong Vessels. It strengthens the Kidneys, fortifies original Qi, warms the Spleen & aids in digestion. It relieves menstrual pain & assists conception by promoting the circulation of Qi & Blood.
Ren 2 - Warms the Uterus
ST-29 - Treats uterine Blood Stasis due to cold. Restores menstruation to normal & warms the Lower Jiao, most particularly the uterus in women. ST-29 is normally treated with warm needling to warm the uterus & drive out pathogenic cold.
DU 4 with Moxa - Tonifies the Kidneys. Expels Cold. Strengthens Jing

BL 23 - Warms the Uterus. Tonifies Jing. Fortifies Kidney Yang
Kid 3 – Strengthens the Kidneys

Other possible endometriosis patterns:

3. Blood Stasis with Liver Qi Stagnation

Signs & Symptoms
- Painful periods with intense, stabbing pain that begin before the menses and persists during menstruation.
- Blood is dark red with large clots.
- Pain relieved after passing clots.
- Blood flow may vary and be either scanty or heavy, accompanied by hypochondrium (upper abdominal) pain.
- PMS symptoms include feelings of depression/becoming easily upset.
- Possible swollen breasts
- Hard and immobile abdominal masses
Tongue: Dark purple or dark reddish tongue with thin white coating
Pulse - Wiry, taut or choppy.
Tx: Sooth the Liver, invigorate the Blood & move stasis to stop pain

Possible Acupuncture Points
Liv 3 – Moves Liver Qi & removes stagnation. Major point to activate the Penetrating Vessel.
LI 4 – Aids in ascending or descending Qi
SP 8 - Regulates menstruation & Invigorates Blood
SP 10 – Moves, cools & tonifies the Blood
Liv 14 – Cools & invigorates the Blood. Treats uterine bleeding.
BL 17 - Moves & cools the Blood
Zi Gong (Palace of the Child) – Regulates menstruation, prolapse of the Uterus & uterine bleeding. Treats lower abdominal pain due to obstruction of Qi & Blood.
BL 32 – Invigorates the Blood. Tonifies the Kidneys. Regulates menstruation & stops leucorrhoea, a thick, whitish or yellowish vaginal discharge. There are many causes of leukorrhea, the usual one being estrogen imbalance.

4. Blood Stasis with Qi & Blood Deficiency

Signs & Symptoms
- Fatigue
- Dizziness
- Painful periods that are worse after the period with lower abdominal dull ache which feels better when pressure is applied.
- Scanty periods with Blood that is light in colour, thin in texture combined with a pale complexion.
- Poor appetite with loose stools.

Tongue: Light coloured with thin white coating
Pulse: Weak & thin.
Tx: Reinforce Qi, nourish Blood & invigorate Qi & Blood to stop pain.

Possible Acupuncture Points
Ren 4 – Regulates the Uterus. Nourishes & builds Blood & tonifies original Qi

Ren 6 - Tonifies upright Qi, Yuan & Yang Qi. Expels dampness. Regulates the circulation of Qi & Blood. With moxa excellent to control diarrhea.

SP 10 - Moves, cools & tonifies Blood. Regulates the circulation of Qi & Blood.

DU 20 – Calms the Spirit. Raises sinking Qi & counters prolapse.

ST 36 – Nourishes Blood. Tonifies Qi & expels Dampness

SP 8 - Regulates menstruation & invigorates Blood

SP 1 – Stops bleeding (Holds Blood in its proper place) & tonifies the Spleen.

Liv 3 – Moves Liver Qi & removes stagnation.

LI 4 – Regulates the upward & downward movement of Qi

5. Blood Stasis with Liver & Kidney Yin Deficiency

Signs & Symptoms
- Painful periods with dull abdominal pain during and after period
- Period bleeding can be heavy or light but is red in colour
- Dizziness
- Tinnitus
- Lower back pain and sore knees
- Blurry vision
- Hair loss

- Poor memory
- Tiredness
Tongue: Light reddish with a thin white tongue coat.
Pulse: Deep, thready & weak
Tx: Nourish Liver Blood & Kidney Yin. Regulate menstruation & Stop pain.

Possible Acupuncture Points
BL 18 (Liver Shu Point) – Regulates & nourishes Liver Blood
BL 23 (Kidney Shu Point) – Nourishes Kidney Yang & Yin Qi. Benefits & warms the Uterus. Builds Blood.
BL 17 – (Diaphragm Shu) – Invigorates & nourishes Blood & dispels Stasis. Cools Blood Heat & stops bleeding. Calms the Spirit.
SP 6 – Meeting point of the three foot Yin meridians. Fortifies the Liver, Spleen & Kidneys helping to regulate Qi & Blood circulation & relieve menstrual pain. Tonifies Kidneys & Yin Qi. Benefits the Uterus. Cools & Invigorates the Blood. Stops bleeding.
Kid 14 (Meeting point of the Kidney channel with the Penetrating vessel) – Regulates Qi & moves Blood. Harmonizes Ren & Chong Mai. Opens waterways.
Kid 3 - Nourishes Kidney Yin & Yang
Liv 8 - Cools, builds & invigorates Blood. Nourishes Liver Yin.
SP 10 - Moves, cools & tonifies Blood
Liv 6 - (Xi-Clef Point) Regulates Blood. (Mainly uterine bleeding). Treats persistent flow of lochia (the normal discharge from the Uterus after childbirth).
LU 9 - Tonifies & nourishes Yin. Calms the pulse.

6. Blood Stasis with Heat in the Blood

Signs & Symptoms
- Painful periods with severe pain
- A hot water bottle will make pain worse
- Pain increases with each cycle and worsens before and during period
- Menstrual bleeding is heavy and the Blood is dark red with clots
- The menstrual cycle will become shorter and shorter, even as little as three weeks.
- PMS symptoms may include becoming easily angered with breast and chest distension, restlessness of Heart (vexation), palpitations, bitter taste and dry mouth.

- May prefer drinking cold water.
Tongue: Red with dry yellow fur
Pulse: Wiry, rapid pulse.
Tx: Clear Heat, cool Blood & regulate menstruation to stop pain.

Possible Acupuncture Points
Liv 1 - Regulates Liver Qi & Stops menstrual bleeding.
Liv 2 - Cools Blood. Clears Liver Fire. Sedates the Liver.
Liv 4 - Clears stagnant Heat from the Liver channel. Regulates Qi in the genitals, urinary system & area below the umbilicus.
Liv 5 - Clears Damp Heat from the Lower Jiao. Major Point for vaginal infections. Regulates menstruations. Benefits the genitals (Itching, pain, swelling, incessant erection, Shan disorder, Plumstone Qi in Lower Abdomen)
SP 6 - Tonifies Kidneys & Yin. Benefits the Uterus. Cools & invigorates the Blood. Stops bleeding.
Kid 2 - Clears false Heat. Cools the Blood. Tonifies the Kidneys.
LI 11 - Clears Heat & cools the Blood.
Ren 3 - Regulates the Uterus & menstruation. Strengthens the Kidneys. Helps with the retention of the placenta. Clears Heat.
BL 32 - Invigorates the Blood. Tonifies the Kidneys. Regulates menstruation & stops leucorrhoea.
DU 14 - Clears Yang Heat. Pacifies Wind.

7. Blood Stasis with Damp Phlegm

Signs & Symptoms
- Painful periods with a dull abdominal ache accompanied with consistent vaginal clear or white discharge
- Period can be delayed or irregular with spotting before or after menses
- Blood flow is dark-brownish with sticky mucus-like clots.
- Fatigue
- Heavy & "muddy" head
- Concentration difficulties
- Poor memory
- Chest stuffiness with phlegm
- Heavy body
- Poor appetite
- Stomach fullness

- Loose stools
- Cloudy urination
Pulse: Soft or slippery
Tongue: Swollen with teeth marks & a greasy, sticky coating.
Tx: Remove Blood Stasis & clear Damp Phlegm by tonifing Spleen Qi.

Possible Acupuncture Points
SP 9 - Resolves Dampness & Phlegm
ST 40 - Resolves Dampness & Phlegm
Ren 3 - Drains Damp Heat. Regulates the Uterus & menstruation. Strengthens the Kidneys. Helps with the retention of the placenta.
Ren 12 - Expels Dampness & tonifies the Spleen
ST 36 - Expels Dampness & tonifies the Spleen. Nourishes Blood. Tonifies Qi.
Ren 17 - Expels Phlegm. Regulates the Qi.
SP 4 - Tonifies the Speen & transforms Dampness.
PC 6 - Balances Yin meridians & Blood. Calms the Spirit.
SP 10 - Moves, cools & tonifies the Blood.
Zi Gong - (Palace of the Child) Infertility. Regulates menstruation. Prolapse of the Uterus. Uterine bleeding. Brings Qi & Blood to the Uterus.
BL 32 - Relieves Blood Stasis. Treats dysmenorrhea & irregular menstruations. Tonifies the Kidneys.

8. Blood Stasis with Damp Heat

With Damp Heat, Dampness is the predominant pathogenic factor. Therefore, in addition to invigorating Blood the focus of treatment is on draining or resolving Dampness.

Signs & Symptoms
- Painful periods with vaginal yellow, sticky and smelly discharge
- Red menstrual Blood with small clots.
- Abdominal pain that is worse during intercourse and especially painful with certain positions.
- Hypogastric pain before the period and sometimes mid cycle
- Burning sensation extending to the sacrum.
- Ultrasound shows "pelvic cavity masses", often accompanied with lower back and lower abdominal pain.
- Dislikes heat and pressure on the abdomen.

- Constipation
- Anus pain from difficult defecation
- Hot or itching sensation in the vaginal area.
- Yellow cloudy urination
- Sticky, smelly stools
- Thirst
- Feeling of Heat

Pulse: Slippery & rapid
Tongue: Reddish with sticky yellow fur.
Tx: Clear Damp Heat & remove Blood Stasis to stop pain.

Possible Acupuncture Points

Liv 2 - Clears fire & moves Liver Qi
Liv 3 - Drains Damp Heat from the Lower Burner. Moves Qi & opens obstructions.
SP 6 - Transforms Dampness & invigorates Blood
SP 9 - Transforms Dampness & drains damp Heat from Lower Burner.
SP 10 - Clears Heat & cools the Blood
SP 13 - Regulates the Qi. Treats abdominal masses & pain.
ST 12 - Clears Heat. Softens masses.
Ren 3 - Drains Damp Heat. Regulates the Uterus.
BL 17 (Diaphragm Shu) - Clears Heat & cools Blood
BL 32 - Invigorates Blood & strengthens the Kidneys
LI 11 - Cools the Blood & drains damp Heat. Softens masses.
DU 14 - Clears Heat. Tonifies Yang Qi.

Ovarian Cysts

An ovarian cyst is a thinned-walled sac filled with fluid that forms on or beside an ovary. Every month the ovaries develop a follicle which normally releases an egg during ovulation. Cysts grow when a follicle grows but neither releases an egg nor degenerates. Instead, it continues to grow in the ovary, secreting fluid that develops into a cyst.

Ovarian cysts can cause menstrual blood stagnation, leading to pain, menstrual irregularities, excessive bleeding, amenorrhea, constipation and infertility. In addition, because stagnation often develops into excess heat, a woman will sometimes suffer from hot flashes, insomnia or a host of inflammatory conditions.

Additional Symptoms:
- Pressure, fullness, heaviness, swelling, or pain in the abdomen
- Pain during period
- Constant pain or burning inside and above the hip bone, or on either side of the lower abdomen
- Sudden twisting movements are painful, and the area is usually very sensitive to touch.
- Dull ache in the lower back and thighs
- Pain during sex
- Weight gain
- Abnormal bleeding
- Nausea or vomiting
- Breast tenderness
- Change in frequency or ease of urination (such as inability to fully empty the bladder)
- Difficulty with bowel movements due to pressure on the adjacent pelvic anatomy
- Fatigue, headaches, nausea or vomiting
Tongue: Swollen with a thick greasy or yellow coating
Pulse: Slippery

If the cause of the cysts is Endometriosis, periods may be heavy, and intercourse painful. If the cause is Polycystic Ovarian Syndrome (PCOS), symptoms may include increased facial hair or body hair, acne, obesity, insulin resistance, and infertility from irregular or absence of ovulation.

PCOS is one of the most common endocrine disorders and a major cause of infertility in women. With PCOS, the cysts and connective tissue surrounding them produce male hormones called androgens which block follicular development preventing the release of mature eggs.

The follicles start to grow but the eggs are not released from the follicles. Some follicles remain as cysts. Progesterone is not produced causing an irregular or complete absence of the menstrual cycle.

Irregular periods may occur 4 to 5 times a year with a heavy Blood flow. Some women do not ovulate and experience little or no bleeding. If an egg is released it is often later in the cycle and lower in quality due to the unhealthy state of the reproductive system.

Many women with PCOS still believe they are ovulating due to positive results from ovulation predictor kits which detect elevated levels of LH caused by the increased presence of estrogen in the Blood.

The Kidneys, Spleen and Liver are all involved in this disorder in addition to a disharmony of the Chong and Ren meridians. From a TCM point of view, cysts are stagnation of Qi and Phlegm, a consequence of water accumulating in the abdominal cavity where it transforms into phlegm, usually because of Kidney Yang Deficiency. There may often be coexisting Blood stagnation or Liver Qi stagnation.

The treatment principle, depending on clinical signs and symptoms, is to tonify Kidney Yang, transform phlegm, move water, dredge or move Liver Qi, invigorate Blood and break Blood Stasis. The main goal of treatment is to induce ovulation by regulating the menstrual cycle.

This approach is performed regardless of the type of cyst, or whether it involves polycystic ovaries. In cases of PCOS, treatment is more complicated and takes longer, but is often treatable.

Chinese herbal medicine is very effective in treating functional ovarian cysts with accumulations of fluid or Blood. A herbal formula used to treat this disorder is Phlegm Transforming Formula or Xia Ku Hua Tan Pian. This formula dissolves phlegm, disperses phlegm nodules, moves Blood, regulates Qi, clears heat toxins, eliminates dampness, nourishes Yin and Blood, and supports the Spleen and Kidneys.

Possible Acupuncture Points
Sp 4 & PC 6, Kid 13, Kid 14, Liv 3 - Opens Chong Mai to reduce Blood Stasis
Lu 7 & Kid 6, Ren 4, St 28, Zi Gong - Opens Ren Mai to Nourish Yin
Si 3 & BL 62, Ren 4 - Opens Du Mai Meridian to Move Blood. Strengthens Kidney Yang
Sp 6, SP 9, Ren 5, Ren 9, St 28, Kid 14 - Opens Waterways. St 28 clears stasis of Qi & Blood from the Uterus.
BL 22 (San Jiao Shu), St 40 - Resolves Damp Phlegm
Kid 3, Kid 13, St 36, BL 23 (Kidney Shu), BL 20 (Spleen Shu), Ren 4 - Strengthens Kidneys & Spleen
Sp 10, PC 6, BL 17 (Diaphragm Shu), **Sp 6, Liv 3, Kid 14** - Resolves Blood Stasis
Liv 2, Liv 3, Liv 8 - Releases Stagnant Liver Qi

The choice of points depends in part on the presenting condition and rhythm of the menstrual cycle. As it takes 100 days for the body to produce a healthy egg, patients should wait for three menstrual cycles before trying to get pregnant.

According to E Douglas Kihn, OMD, LAc, of Acupuncture Today, electro-acupuncture can be an effective tool in treating cysts. First, determine exactly where the cyst lies, either by palpation, from the location of the patient's pain, or from information supplied by her gynecologist.

Then, have her lie on her side so that you can place needles in the abdominal and low back in areas that will allow electrical current to run directly through the growth, being careful not to cross the mid-line of the body. Treat for thirty minutes. Do not use electro-acupuncture during the Luteal Phase after ovulation.

Supplement the treatment by needling tender Liver and Gall Bladder points especially on the feet and legs. Common points are **Liv 3, GB 41, and Liv 8**. In addition, **SP 9 and ST 40** will help reduce stagnation of Dampness and Phlegm.

Auricular Acupuncture: Treat reactive points in the ear-Uterus area, situated in the anterior corner of the triangular fossa.

Uterine Fibroids (Myomas)

Fibroids are non-cancerous tumors that grow mostly in the muscular wall and connective tissue of the Uterus. Another medical term for fibroids is myoma. Fibroids depend on estrogen and progesterone to grow so normally they will shrink after the onset of menopause.

Fibroids are found in approximately 20% of women over 35 years of age. They can grow as a single or multiple tumor. They can be as small as an apple seed or as big as a grapefruit. Some lesions may spread towards the outside of the Uterus or towards the internal abdominal cavity.

Signs & Symptoms

Most fibroids, particularly when small, do not cause any symptoms but some women with fibroids can experience:
- Heavy abdominal bleeding or painful periods
- Feeling of fullness in the pelvic area (lower stomach area)
- Enlargement of the lower abdomen
- Frequent and urgent urination or incontinence
- Bowel difficulties (particularly constipation)
- Pain during sex
- Lower back pain
- Severe menstrual pain and flooding

Symptoms depend on the location of the lesion and its size. While fibroids are common, they are not normally a cause of infertility accounting for about 3% of reasons why a woman may not conceive.

Nevertheless, fibroids may hinder conception by blocking the uterine cavity or the entrance into the uterus from the fallopian tubes. They can also block the embryo from implanting in the uterus wall.

Complications are possible during pregnancy and labor such as a six-time greater risk of miscarriage, bleeding, premature labor and caesarean section due to a lack of room in the Uterus or birth canal caused by the presence of the fibroid or fibroids.

According to Traditional Chinese Medicine (TCM), the appearance of fibroids is characterized as fixed masses in the Uterus caused by the stagnation of Qi and uterine Blood. In some cases, accumulation of Phlegm plays a secondary role.

As a result, the menstrual cycle becomes blocked, obstructing the normal reproductive rhythm. Stagnation of Qi and uterine Blood can result from emotional issues, from the accumulation of Cold, or from exposure to Dampness in the lower abdomen.

The most important factor affecting this condition is the invasion of the lower abdomen by Cold, which impairs the proper circulation of Qi and Blood eventually leading to Blood Stasis and the formation of masses. Cold pathogenic factors are aggravated by exposure to cold or raw foods or to a cold environment.

Uterine fibroids are related to an imbalance in the Liver and Spleen. Pathogenic Cold, Dampness, Heat or toxins that remain in the body for a long time impair the functions of these organs causing Qi, Blood and/or Phlegm stagnation.

External Dampness may also invade the meridians of the legs settling in the lower abdomen transforming into Phlegm and eventually into abdominal masses. Damp pathogenic factors are aggravated by excessive consumption of greasy foods or dairy products.

The treatment is like the approach recommended for endometriosis and, as usual, follows the pattern differentiation established according to the signs and symptoms of the individual patient.

Acupuncture, Chinese herbs, abdominal massage, topical herbal applications, dietary regulation, and exercise including Qi Gong are all useful in the treatment of fibroids. Treatment involves invigorating the Blood and eliminating Blood Stasis, moving the Qi, clearing Heat, and softening the hardened masses and surrounding tissue. If there are signs of accumulation of Damp, the treatment plan may include supplementing Spleen Qi.

Giovanni Maciocia, author and world-renowned acupuncturist believes that endometriosis treatments protocols applied to fibroids can be helpful but are less effective. In addition, according to Maciocia Chinese Medicine can only treat small fibroids that are 2 to 3 cm in size.

Therefore, the therapist must know the size of the fibroid before undertaking treatment. If the fibroid is bigger than 2 to 3 cm a combination of acupuncture and herbs may still have a positive effect and, at a minimum, may help reduce bleeding which is a major symptom if this condition.

It normally takes a minimum of three menstrual cycles to regulate the movement of Blood. When Uterine fibroids are the main issue, the treatment may take considerably longer.

In Traditional Chinese Medicine, abdominal masses are divided into two categories, Qi masses and Blood masses. A contemporary Chinese physician, Professor Shen Zhong-Li, has found that Uterine Fibroids represent as stagnation of Qi and Blood caused by a combination of Spleen and Stomach deficiency and Liver constraint or Fire leading to a gradual loss of function in the extraordinary vessels. (Source: Acupuncture Wellness Center of New Orleans, LA)

Professor Shen categorizes women suffering from fibroids into three major patterns: Qi and Blood Stagnation, Yin Deficiency with Fire, and Liver Qi Stagnation with Spleen Qi Deficiency.

General Treatment Points
Sp 6, Sp 8, Sp 10, BL 17 – Invigorate Blood to resolve Blood Stasis
Kid 3, Kid 7- Increase Blood circulation to the reproductive organs
Liv 2, Liv 3, Liv 8 - Help to detoxify any excess hormones. Resolve Qi stagnation & invigorate the Blood

1. Qi Stagnation and Blood Stasis

Qi stagnation is often brought on by emotional stress. Both Qi Stagnation and Blood Stasis may be a result of physical trauma as in a major surgery, a significant injury or even a difficult childbirth. Blood stasis can be caused by abnormally heavy bleeding with menses, excessive sexual activity or having sex while menstruating.

Signs & Symptoms
- Normally the patient has a regular menstrual cycle
- In severe cases damage to the Penetrating and Conception Vessels may lead to heavy periods.
- Scanty but long-lasting menstrual bleeding
- Menstrual Blood often dark with clots if Blood Stasis predominant
- Lower abdominal distension
- Latent pain and a dragging sensation in the rectum

Tongue: Tends to be dark red & the sides may show purple spots.
Pulse: Deep & wiry, or thin & choppy.
Tx: Move Qi & Blood. Eliminate Stasis. Stop pain.

Possible Acupuncture Points
Sp 4 & PC 6 - Opens the Chong Mai. Moves Blood.
Liv 3 - Regulates the Liver. Moves Qi. Invigorates the Blood.
GB 34 - Moves Liver Qi. Removes stagnation.
SP 10 - Cools, Moves & Builds Blood
BL 17 (Diaphragm Shu) - Cools, Moves & Builds Blood
Kid 14 - Regulates Qi, Blood & the Triple Burner
Sp 6 - Builds & Invigorates Blood
Sp 8 - Help to resolve Blood stasis. Transforms Dampness.
Lu 7 & Kid 6 with Ren 6 – Tonifies the Uterus & Ovaries. Moves Qi in the Lower Abdomen
Zi Gong - Brings Qi & Blood to the Uterus. Regulates menstruation.

2. Kidney & Liver Yin Deficiency with Empty Fire Blazing

This is an advanced stage of Yin Deficiency from a Deficiency of Kidney Qi or a chronic illness. Occurs when the body is most deficient.

Signs & Symptoms
- Menstruations tend to be early & heavy or scanty but with long-lasting bleeding and possibly trickling after menses
- After the period blood-streaked white discharge or yellow-white vaginal discharge
- Menstrual Blood is red or scarlet red
- Mid-cycle bleeding
- Menstruations often accompanied by a burning sensation in the chest or a feeling of heat in the lower abdomen

- Pain in the nipples
- Sensation of itching in the breast, or even a stabbing pain and distension and pain in the entire breast before the period.
- Malar flush, nights sweats, dry mouth and throat at night. Insomnia.
Tongue: Red with little moisture & the tongue coat will be reduced or thin yellow.
Pulse: Wiry & thin, thin, fine & rapid or floating, empty pulse.
Tx: Nourish Yin to benefit Kidneys. Nourish the Liver

Possible Acupuncture Points
LU 7 on the left **& Kid 6** on the right - Opens Ren Mai. Nourishes Kidney Yin.
Kid 12 - Tonifies Kidneys & Yuan Qi. Harmonizes Ren & Chong Mai
Ren 4 - Supports the Uterus & Blood. Tonifies Yang & Yin Qi.
HE 6 - Clears False Heat. Nourishes Yin.
Kid 3 - Tonify Kidneys. Nourishes Kidney Yin. Clears deficiency Heat.
Ren 7 - Tonifies the Kidneys & Yin Qi. Benefits the genital region.
SP 6 - Nourishes Yin. Tonifies the Spleen.
LI 11, Kid 2, Liv 2, Liv 3, SP 6, SP 10, & PC 3 – All points cool Blood & remove stasis.
ST 36 - Tonifies the Kidneys, Liver and Spleen. Nourishes Liver Blood in gynecological conditions.
Liv 8 - Nourishes & invigorates Blood. Sedates the Liver. Nourishes the Kidneys

3. Damp Heat from Liver Qi Stagnation with Spleen Qi Deficiency

The origin of this pattern is usually Liver constraint and Spleen Qi Deficiency. The Spleen is therefore unable to transform Qi and Blood into menstrual Blood. Damp accumulations congeal from Liver Heat, producing substantial phlegm, in the form of uterine fibroids.

Fibroid tumors often form soft mass fibroids or myomas. Patients present with mixed deficient and excess patterns that change from predominant excess at the onset of the disorder to increasing deficiency. The pattern is difficult to treat.

Signs & Symptoms
- Menstrual cycle tends to be normal or late with heavy bleeding often accompanied by small red clots.

- Pulling down sensation in the lower abdomen
- Loose stools or diarrhea and/or other digestive problems
- Thin or excessive vaginal discharge following menstruation
- Oppression of the chest
- Scanty dark urine
- Breast nodules
- Overweight
- Post-nasal drip

Tongue: Tongue body tends to be swollen with a sticky white fur that may be thick or thin.

Pulse: Slippery & thin or thin & wiry.

Tx: Clear Heat & Resolve Dampness to eliminate Stasis, resolving Dampness being the priority for treatment.

Possible Acupuncture Points

Lu 7 Right **& Kid 6** Left - Opens Ren Channel. Nourishes Yin.

GB 41 Right & **SJ 5** Left - Regulates the Girdle Vessel & drains dampness.

Ren 3 & Zi Gong (3 cun lateral to Ren 3) Bilateral - Strengthens the Uterus & removes dampness.

St 28, BL 22, Ren 5 - Opens waterways. Clears Dampness in the Lower Burner.

SP 3, SP 6, SP 9, ST 40 – Resolves Dampness & Phlegm

St 30 & Kid 14 (Pts of intersection with Chong) - Eliminates stagnation in the Penetrating Vessel.

Liv 3, GB 34, GB 41 - Moves Liver Qi & removes stagnation

ST 36 – Transforms Dampness. Nourishes Yin. Tonifies Spleen Qi.

Pelvic Inflammatory Disease (PID)

PID is a major cause of infertility. It is an infection or inflammation of the female pelvic organ and/or connective tissues that can permanently scar the reproductive tract and lead to female infertility. It's usually caused by a sexually transmitted infection (STI) like chlamydia or gonorrhea and is treated with antibiotics.

Some possible causes of PID are the presence of foreign objects in the Uterus, including Intra Uterine Devices (IUDs), pelvic region surgeries including abortions, which may involve infectious complications, appendicitis and infections of the Urinary Bladder and Large Intestine. Early on there may be no noticeable symptoms of PID. Some patients report no symptoms or intermittent symptoms. But as the infection gets worse, the patient may experience:

- Pain in your lower abdomen and pelvis
- Heavy discharge from the vagina with an unpleasant odor
- Irregular menstrual bleeding, bleeding between periods or pain
- Pain during sex
- Fever and chills
- Painful or difficult urination
- Nausea or vomiting

Acupuncture and herbal medicine have long been used to resolve chronic pelvic region infections. In Chinese medicine, PID is classified as the invasion of Damp Heat and Toxins causing Qi and Blood Stasis in the Lower Burner affecting the Liver channel and the Belt Vessel.

According to TCM, the primary symptoms, particularly of acute PID, are leukorrhea and lower abdominal pain. The acute stage involves Heat more than Damp and the chronic stage involves Damp more than Heat.

Deficiency syndromes often complicate this diagnosis when PID becomes chronic. To help identify the nature of the disorder, ask questions related to the discharge, as well as to the location and type of pain experienced by the patient.

Most cases of PID involve abnormal vaginal discharge. A profuse and watery discharge without any smell or irritation points to accumulatio of Damp and Cold. A pus-like, discolored and foul-smelling discharge that causes irritation, itching or burning points to Damp Heat.

Acupuncture will increase the immune system's ability to fight the infection, decrease inflammation in the reproductive tract, reduce pain and help prevent adhesions and scarring in the pelvic cavity.

Tx: Resolve Dampness, clear Heat, strengthen the immune system, reduce inflammation, and encourage Blood flow.

Possible Acupuncture Points
GB 41 & SJ 5 with GB 26 - Opens Belt Vessel. Drains Dampness.
Ren 4 - Tonifies Original Qi. Builds Blood & Yin. Regulates the Uterus. Treats vaginal discharge & abdominal pain.
Ren 6 - Tonifies Original Qi. Generates Qi & Yang. Expels Dampness. Invigorates Blood. Treats vaginal discharge & abdominal pain.
SP 6 - Transforms Dampness. Invigorates & cools Blood. Tonifies Spleen & Kidneys.
ST 29 - Warms the Uterus & drives out Cold. Invigorates Blood. Promotes Urination. Treats lower abdominal pain.
SP 10 - Clears Heat. Cools Blood.
ST 25 (Large Intestine Mu Point) - Clears Dampness & damp Heat. Eliminates stasis in Lower Abdomen.
Zi Gong - Regulates menstruation & alleviates pain.

For patients with Blood Stasis
LV 5 - Invigorates Blood & moves Qi
SP 9 - Drains damp Heat from Lower Burner. Treats abdominal pain.

For patients with Qi Deficiency & Blood Stasis
ST 36 - Clears Fire. Expels Dampness. Tonifies Original Qi.
Kid 3 - Nourishes Essence & Kidney Yin & Yang Qi. Clears Deficiency Heat.

Additional Points
Ren 3 - Drains Damp Heat. Regulates the Uterus. Tonifies the Kidneys.
ST 28 - Regulates water passages. Tonifies the Kidneys.
Kid 7 - Drains Damp Heat. Tonifies the Kidneys.

BL 23 (Kidney Shu Point) - Tonifies Original Qi & strengthens Kidneys Yin & Yang. Warms & benefits the Uterus.

Acupuncture therapy can be applied 3 times per week for 3 months. Needling technique is reinforcing and reducing until sense of de Qi is felt. After sense of de Qi has arrived, the needle will stay at its place for thirty minutes during which the acupuncture needles may be manipulated once. A heat lamp can be applied to warm the abdomen.

Counter Indicated Points for Pregnancy

Points	Effect
LI 4	Causes Qi to descend & induces labor
SP 6	May induce labor - Uterine contraction
GB 21	Do not use until after 34 weeks due to its ability to descend Qi
Points on the Sacrum **BL 31, BL 32, (BL 33, BL 34)**	Tendency to induce labour
BL 60	Promotes labour
BL 67	May induce labour
Points between the umbilicus and the pubis	Risk of needling too deep.
Lu 7 right, **Kid 6** left	Opens the Ren Channel
Points above the umbilicus after 3 months of pregnancy	An increased likelihood this style of treatment may cause contractions.
No strong or tonifying treatments (especially of the back) between weeks 32 & 34	Causes the fetus to descend.

Full, Empty and Damp Heat

Heat (Excess Yang)

Diet of fried foods, alcohol, an external pathogenic factor that penetrates the interior of the body and emotional stress can lead to the appearance of Heat.

Signs & Symptoms
- Agitation
- Anxiety
- Insomnia with nightmares
- Feeling of heat
- Red face or head
- Constipation (Dry Stools)
- Desire for cold drinks
- Scanty dark urine
- Thirst

Tongue: Red, dry, with yellow coat
Pulse: Rapid, full

Generally, to clear Full or Empty Heat, use Fire Points such as:
PC 8 - Clears Heat from the Pericardium & Heart. Cools the Blood. Calms the Spirit
HT 8 - Clears Heart Fire. Calms the Spirit.
Liv 2 - Clears Liver Fire. Cools the Blood. Pacifies Liver Wind.
LU 10 - Clears Heat from the Lungs. Tonifies & calms agitation of the Heart. Descends rebellious Qi from the upper body. Harmonizes the Stomach & the Heart.
Kid 2 - Clears false Heat. Cools the Blood. Tonifies the Kidneys.
SP 2 - Clears Dampness & Damp Heat. Tonifies the Spleen.

The treatment varies depending on which organ system is involved.

Other points to clear Heat:
LI 11 - Clears Heat & damp Heat. Cools the Blood. Softens masses.
DU 14 - Calms the Spirit. Clears Yang Heat. Expels Wind.
ST 36 - Clears Fire. Expels Dampness. Builds Blood.
SJ 6 - Clears Heat in 3 Jiaos. Softens masses.

ST 41 - Clears Heat. Treats vertigo, dizziness & fever.
SP 10 - Clears Heat & cools the Blood
Kid 6 - Calms the Spirit. Cools the Blood. Malar flush. Vaginal infections.

Empty Heat

Empty Heat derives from Yin deficiency. According to Giovanni Maciocia, the term Empty Heat may give the impression that Empty Heat is not real Heat. Although deriving from Yin deficiency, Empty Heat is real Heat and it heats up as much as Full Heat.

The second important clarification is that, although Empty Heat derives from Yin deficiency, it may occur by itself for years before giving rise to Empty Heat. Although Empty Heat derives from Yin deficiency, it takes time for it to develop. Therefore, one may have Yin deficiency for years without Empty Heat.

The tongue shows this very clearly. Yin deficiency manifests on the tongue with lack of coating. If there is Yin deficiency without Empty Heat, the tongue will lack a coating but will have a normal colour.

Signs & Symptoms
- Feeling of heat in the afternoon/evening
- Dry mouth with desire to drink in small sips
- Malar flush (red cheekbones)
- Dry throat at night
- Feeling of heat in the chest, palms & soles (also called 5-Palm Heat)
- Dry stools
- Scanty-dark urine
Pulse: Floating, Empty & Rapid
Tongue: Red tongue without coating.

To subdue and clear Empty Heat needle:
LI 4 - Clears Heat from the head. (Can educe labour & promote expulsion of dead fetus)
PC 7 - Clears Heat. Cools the Blood. Calms the Spirit. Eases emotional separation.
& HT 6 - Clears False Heat. Nourishes Yin. Tonifies the Heart. Calms the Spirit.

Kid 2 – Clears false Heat.

To clear Empty Heat, one must also nourish Yin.

To nourish Yin:
SP 6 - Supplements Yin. Tonifies the Spleen. Transforms Dampness.
Ren 12 (Stomach Mu Point) - Tonifies the Spleen. Expels Dampness.
Kid 3 - Supplements Kidney Yin & clears deficiency Heat
Kid 6 - Supplements Kidney Yin & clears deficiency Heat.

Generally, one can use the Yuan Source Points of the Yin organs to nourish Yin such as:
Liv 3 - Nourishes Liver Blood & Liver Yin
LU 9 - Nourishes Yin. Tonifies Lung Qi & Yin. Calms the pulse.

Damp Heat

Dampness is the predominant factor. Concentrate on draining or resolving Dampness rather than clearing Heat. Dampness is sticky, it lingers, is heavy and difficult to get rid of. It slows things down, infuses downwards and causes repeated attacks.
To treat, focus on stimulating the movement, transformation and excretion of fluids in each of the Three Burners.

Upper Burner: DU 26, LU 7, LI 4, LI 6, SJ 4, SJ 6, REN 17
Middle Burner: REN 9, REN 11, REN 12, ST 22
Lower Burner: ST 28, BL 22, REN 5, BL 39, SP 6, SP 9, KID 7
Phlegm Heat: ST 40 & PC 5

References

- Obstetrics and Gynecology in Chinese Medicine by Giovanni Maciocia, Second Edition, Churchill, Livingston, Elsevier
- College of Acupuncture and Therapeutics
- A Manual of Acupuncture by Peter Deadman
- Chinese Medical Qi Gong by Tianjun Liu, O.M.D.
- Encyclopedia of Natural Healing by Siegfried Gursche, MH
- Infertility: Using Chinese Herbal medicine to Promote Fertility and Prevent Miscarriage by Jake Paul Fratkin, OMD, L.Ac.
- St. John, Meredith: New England School of Acupuncture, Etiology and Pathology Lecture Notes
- Valaskatgis, Peter: New England School of Acupuncture, Etiology and Pathology Lecture Notes
- How Acupuncture Enhances Fertility by Robin Hays, LAc, OMD and Nancy Rakela, LAc, OMD, Gerhard and Postneck, 1992
- Influence of Acupuncture on the pregnancy rate in patients who undergo ART. Fertility & Sterility Vol77 April 2002
- Reduction of Blood flow impedance in the uterine arteries of infertile women with Electro Acupuncture, Stener-Victirin, et al., Human Reproduction, Vol 11, no6. pp. 1311-17, 1996
- Clinical Guide to Commonly Used Herbal Formulas by John Scott, Lorena Monda & John Heuertz, Herbal Medicine Press 2014
- The Infertility Cure by Randine Lewis, Ph.D., Master of Science in Oriental Medicine. Little, Brown and Company, 2004
- Treatment of Infertility with Chinese Medicine, Jane Lyttleton, BSc, MPhil, Dip TCM, Certified Acupuncturist & Herbal Medicine, Churchill, Livingstone, Elsevier, 2013

- wikipedia.org
- adeinstitute.com
- babyzone.com
- pacificcollege.edu
- iaac.ca/en
- somaacupuncture.com

- YinYanghouse.com
- hopkinsmedicine.org
- patient.co.uk
- eugin.co.uk
- healthycanadians.gc.ca
- wellwomanacu.com

- healthcommunities.com
- giovanni-maciocia.com
- jadeinstitute.com
- sacredlotus.com
- americanpregnancy.org
- pacificcollege.edu
- womenshealth.org
- acupuncturetoday.com
- acatcm.com
- medicinenet.com
- attainfertility.com
- webmd.com
- easterncurrents.ca
- acufinder.com
- acupuncturemoxibustion.com
- healthcmi.com
- nurtureacupuncture.com
- differencebetween.com
- nichd.nih.gov
- webmd.com
- londonacupuncturespace.com
- babycenter.com
- plannedparenthood.org
- acupuncturistaustin.com
- simcoehealth.ca
- acufertility.com
- natural-fertility-info.com
- eatright.org
- parenting.com
- choicesmarkets.com
- carahealth.com
- fertilitysmarts.com
- carolinasnaturalhealth.com

- lok-kwan.com
- avicenna.co.uk
- jadeinstitute.com
- draxe.com/irregular-periods
- everydayhealth.com
- yinovacenter.com
- womens-health.co.uk
- acubalance.ca
- natural-fertility-info.com
- nolaacupuncture.com
- medicaldaily.com
- tcmpage.com
- mayoclinic.org
- acupuncture.com
- medical-dictionary.
  thefreedictionary.com
- healthcmi.com
- raeghansiemens.com
- manhattanmidwife.com
- houseoffertilityandhealing.com
- pregnancy.com.au
- vitalitymagazine.com
- mayoclinic.org
- healthnutritionandexercise.com
- journalofchinesemedicine.com
- kindara.com
- dralisonhunter.com
- pregnancy-baby-care.com
- healing-traditions.com
- yinovacenter.com
- chinesemedicineclinic.com
- zoombaby.co.uk

Nourish the Soil
Before Planting the Seed

Old Chinese Saying